Praise for John Robbins and *No Happy Cows*

"John Robbins has inspired a revolution, plain and simple. He saw things that were wrong in the food industry long before any of us did, and with his brilliant research and compelling insight, caused a seismic shift in the way we Americans behold our dinner plates. This book is not only clarifying in terms of the physical, environmental, and spiritual effects of food, but it is inspiring enough to cause material change."

—KATHY FRESTON, *New York Times* bestselling author of *Quantum Wellness* and *Veganist*

"With his singular talent for telling us what we need to know in a way that makes us want to hear it, John Robbins gives us *No Happy Cows*—as engaging as it is informative, and more important than you'll know until you've read it."

—VICTORIA MORAN, author of *Main Street Vegan*

"In this comprehensive yet highly accessible book, John Robbins puts to rest many of the most hotly debated and pressing issues of the times regarding our food choices. With his characteristic grace, compassion, and wisdom, Robbins debunks the myths that have confounded consumers, causing them to act against their own interests and the interests of the planet. This book is a must-read for anyone who cares about their own wellbeing and the wellbeing of the world."

—MELANIE JOY, PhD, EdM, auth3or of *Why We Love Dogs, Eat Pigs, and Wear Cows·* ~~Introduction to Carnism~~

"Every so often, I come across a book of substance—a masterpiece that enriches all aspects of my life. It's rare, but when it happens, I am over the moon. John's new book, *No Happy Cows*, is that kind of book, which I am highly recommending in my work and books. If you wish to upgrade your diet, lose weight, reboot your health, and enhance your life physically, mentally, emotionally, and spiritually, *No Happy Cows* will be your godsend. Every page of this book is filled with food for thought. I encourage you to get several extra copies to keep on hand and give for gifts. It's a must-read for anyone interested in vibrant health from an outstanding author who writes from the heart. Kudos to John Robbins for another life-changing book!"

—SUSAN SMITH JONES, PhD, author of *The Joy Factor* and *Walking on Air*

"John Robbins is one of the most important voices in America today, and the most powerfully sane man I know. He cuts through nonsense like no one else does. He delivers crucial information like no one else does. He gives hope like no one else does. His words are lifelines for the mind, heart, body and soul. When the going gets rough, Robbins' wisdom is what people need to see them through."

—MARIANNE WILLIAMSON, author of *A Return to Love* and *A Woman's Worth*

"John Robbins is the leading voice in the world for restoring humanity to its proper relationship with food, the Earth, and health."

—PAUL HAWKEN, author of *Natural Capitalism*

"A person who leads me to eat in a way that cultivates spiritual awareness is my kind of prophet. John Robbins gives me a light at the end of the tunnel as well as providing a moral compass. The truth has few allies these days. I have deep and abiding respect for John Robbins."

—WOODY HARRELSON, actor and activist

"With regard to our health and the health of our planet, *The Food Revolution* could be the most important book ever written."

—NEALE DONALD WALSCH, author of *Conversations with God*

"John Robbins connects the dots that need connecting—environment, personal health, societal economics, and personal meaning. Scientific researchers also would do well to read what Robbins says."

> —T. COLIN CAMPBELL, author of *The China Study;* professor
> emeritus, Cornell University

"If every patient in every doctor's office read *The Food Revolution*, it would revolutionize the health of America."

> —NEAL BARNARD, MD, president, Physicians Committee
> for Responsible Medicine

"John Robbins provides both the information and the encouragement we need in order to reclaim the health of our bodies and our planet. Packed with political dynamite, *The Food Revolution* will change your life. A must read for everyone who eats."

> —JOANNA MACY, author of *Coming Back to Life* and *Active
> Hope: How to Face the Mess We're in without Going Crazy*

"John Robbins enables us to find our way through the maze of information about food choices and the food industry. His impeccable research and visionary outlook are a gift to those of us who wish to make wise food choices."

> —ANN MORTIFEE, vocal artist and composer

NO HAPPY COWS

Also by John Robbins

*The Food Revolution: How Your Diet Can Help Save Your
Life and Our World*

*The New Good Life: Living Better Than Ever
in an Age of Less*

*Healthy at 100: How You Can—at Any Age—Dramatically
Increase Your Life Span and Your
Health Span*

*Diet for a New America: How Your Food Choices Affect Your
Health, Happiness, and the Future of Life on Earth*

*Reclaiming Our Health: Exploding the Medical Myth and
Embracing the Sources of True Healing*

May All Be Fed: Diet for a New World

The Awakened Heart (with Ann Mortifee)

NO HAPPY COWS

Dispatches from the Frontlines of the Food Revolution

JOHN ROBBINS

AUTHOR OF

The Food Revolution

First published in 2012 by Conari Press, an imprint of
Red Wheel/Weiser, LLC
With offices at:
665 Third Street, Suite 400
San Francisco, CA 94107
www.redwheelweiser.com

ISBN: 978-1-57324-575-3

Library of Congress Cataloging-in-Publication Data
Robbins, John.
No happy cows : dispatches from the frontlines of the food revolution /
John Robbins.
p. cm.
Includes bibliographical references and index.
ISBN 978-1-57324-575-3 (alk. paper)
1. Food habits—United States. 2. Food industry and trade—United
States. 3. Meat industry and trade—United States. 4. Food contami-
nation—United States. 5. Food adulteration and inspection—United
States. 6. Animal welfare—United States. I. Title.

TX371.R634 2012
394.1'20973--dc23

        2011053160

Cover design by Stewart Williams
Cover photograph © Mary R. Vogt/morgue files
Interior by Maureen Forys, Happenstance Type-O-Rama
Typeset in Janson Text with Gotham HTF

Printed in the United States of America
MAL

10 9 8 7 6 5 4 3 2 1

The paper used in this publication meets the minimum requirements
of the American National Standard for Information Sciences—Perma-
nence of Paper for Printed Library Materials Z39.48-1992 (R1997).

Contents

Introduction . . . . *xi*

Part One: Caring for All Creatures

1 The Metamorphosis of a Pig Farmer 3

2 Eggs and the Chickens Who Lay Them 17

3 No Such Thing as Happy Cows 21

Part Two: What Are We Putting into Our Bodies?

4 Health Food or Harm Food? The Truth about Soy . 31

5 Does Soy Cause Alzheimer's? 60

6 It's Not about Size, It's about Health:
   Obesity and Food Choices 67

7 The Skinny on Grass-fed Beef 74

8 Are Factory Farms Becoming Biological
   Weapons Factories? 89

9 Greed and Salmonella: A Deadly Duo 95

10 Infants Growing Breasts: The Trouble with
   Hormones in Our Milk 100

11 Is Your Favorite Ice Cream Made with
   Monsanto's Artificial Hormones? 104

12 The Startling Health Benefits of Dark Chocolate. . 109

Part Three: Industrial Food Production—and Other Dirty Dealings

13 No Sweetness Here: Chocolate and
21st-Century Slavery. 115

14 Bitter Beans: Why Fair Trade Coffee
Matters So Much. 128

15 Pink KFC Buckets? 132

16 Super Size Me. 138

17 The Battle for Our Children 142

18 The Vitaminwater Deception 147

Part Four: Being Human in This Troubled World

19 Remembering How Much Relationships Matter . 153

20 Do Friends Let Friends Eat Junk Food? 158

21 Mike. 162

22 On Suffering 166

23 Stronger at the Broken Places 170

Further Reading and Other Resources *175*

About the Author *183*

John Robbins' Website *185*

Introduction

IT CAN FEEL LIKE A WAR OUT THERE. Who would have guessed that First Lady Michelle Obama was doing anything offensive when, shortly after her husband became president, she planted an organic garden on the White House lawn? It seemed innocuous, much like Lady Bird Johnson's campaign to beautify the nation's cities and highways by planting wildflowers, or Laura Bush's support for childhood literacy.

But CropLife America, a trade association representing Monsanto and other makers of pesticides and genetically modified (GMO) food, was outraged. They angrily wrote the First Lady and widely broadcast their view that her organic garden was unfairly maligning chemical agriculture. They demanded that she use "crop-protection technologies," otherwise known as pesticides.

From the degree of umbrage they took, you'd have thought the Obama administration was nursing major plans to do something to challenge agribusiness as usual. But that was far from the case. In fact, the president had already appointed an ardent ally of industrial agriculture, Tom Vilsack, to head the Department of Agriculture. Vilsack's support for agrichemicals, large industrial farms, and GMO foods was so steadfast that, as the governor of Iowa, he had been the recipient of Monsanto's Governor of the Year award.

As if to make it copiously clear that he was not intending to confront the agrichemical and factory-farm conglomerates, Obama had even appointed the man most responsible for the advancement of GMO food in the history of the U.S., Michael R. Taylor, as senior advisor to the FDA commissioner. And in case that wasn't enough, Obama then promoted Taylor to an even more powerful position as Deputy Commissioner of Foods.

This was the same Michael R. Taylor who had made it possible for Monsanto to get GMO foods approved in the U.S. without even remotely adequate testing for possible health dangers. In a classic example of the "revolving door" between agribusiness and government, Taylor was first an attorney at Monsanto, then became policy chief at the FDA, then became Monsanto's vice president and chief lobbyist, and then was appointed by Obama as America's food-safety czar.

But CropLife America, whose members include such bastions of corporate virtue as Monsanto, Syngenta, DuPont, and Dow, was still not satisfied. In what may have been the political equivalent of make-up sex, the president subsequently appointed CropLife America vice president Islam A. Siddiqui to become the nation's Chief Agricultural Negotiator. Siddiqui is not exactly what you would call a hero to the organic food movement. Nor has he made it his mission to defend future generations and the biological carrying capacity of the planet. When he oversaw the release of the National Organic Program's standards for organic food labeling, it was his bright idea to permit both irradiated and GMO foods to be labeled as organic.

This is the kind of thing, frankly, that makes me upset. It's not a pretty sight to see our nation's food policies in the hands of shills for industrial food production and agrichemical companies like Monsanto. Pesticides in the food chain and in the environment are known to cause cancer, birth defects, autism, and many other ailments. The health effects of GMO foods are largely unknown because there has never been sufficient testing, but what there has been is more frightening than reassuring. A diet based on industrial fast food is contributing mightily to escalating rates of heart disease, obesity, diabetes, and cancer. And factory farms are contributing massively to global warming, deforestation, and species extinction.

Would it be such a terrible idea if, instead of agribusiness as usual, we were to promote sustainable local food systems as a way to rebuild rural economies and improve access to healthy food? Would it be so awful if we were to support family farms rather than factory farms?

Factory farms, also called "confined animal-feeding operations" (CAFOs), now produce almost all of the nation's beef, pork, chicken, dairy, and eggs, but they haven't achieved this level of prominence through rational planning, or efficiencies of scale, or market forces. The factory meat industry has come to dominate the marketplace as the result of federal farm policies that have shifted billions of dollars in environmental, health, and economic costs onto taxpayers and communities. For example, taxpayer-subsidized grain prices save feedlot operations billions of dollars a year in animal feed, while grass-fed beef operations do not benefit at all from this subsidy. The USDA similarly provides billions of our dollars to address factory-farm pollution problems, which wouldn't exist if these operations didn't confine tens of thousands of animals in small areas—a practice that causes great suffering to the animals involved, as well as massive pollution and well-documented health hazards to humans.

What would happen if we had food and agriculture policies that sought to benefit the environment, public health, and rural communities rather than serve industrial agribusiness? What if we made factory farms, rather than taxpayers, pay to prevent or clean up the pollution they create? What if we subsidized healthy foods rather than unhealthy ones?

The health consequences of current policies are now a matter of record. We have the distinction of having become the fattest major nation in the history of the world and, with each passing year, we are becoming noticeably fatter. In 1996, the U.S. already had the highest rate of obesity in the world, but not a single state had an obesity rate higher than 20 percent. By 2011, there was not a single state with an obesity rate lower than 20 percent.

The U.S. now spends far more on healthcare than any other nation. No one else even comes close. Per capita, we spend close to double the amount spent in countries that—other than us—spend the most (Germany, Canada, Denmark, and France).

The annual health insurance premiums paid by the average American family now exceed the gross yearly income of a full-time minimum-wage worker. Every thirty seconds, someone in the U.S. files for bankruptcy due to the costs of treating a health problem.

Healthcare spending is so far out of control that, not only individuals and families, but the entire economy is buckling under the strain. The chairman of Starbucks, Howard Schultz, says his company spends more money on insurance for its employees than it spends on coffee.

And the situation is not improving. A 2011 report found healthcare costs for a typical American family of four had doubled in fewer than nine years.

Have you noticed that in all the heated debate about healthcare reform, one basic fact is rarely discussed—the one thing that could dramatically bring down the costs of healthcare while improving the health of our people? Studies have shown that the single most effective step most people can take to improve their health is to eat a healthier diet. The Centers for Disease Control and Prevention (CDC) estimates that 75 percent of U.S. healthcare spending goes to treat chronic diseases, most of which are preventable and linked to the food we eat. This includes heart disease, stroke, type-2 diabetes, and possibly a third of all cancers.

But isn't this an issue of personal responsibility, you may ask? Isn't it true that what people eat is their own choice? This is true, and it is important. Each of us needs to be accountable for the foods we choose to buy and consume. The government has no business dictating what people should eat. But that is only half of the story. We also have to limit the power that corporations have to influence government policy, for all too often they use that power to maximize their short-term interests and to diminish or eliminate regulations that would protect workers, animals, the environment, and consumers. These same corporations, it should be noted, with all their complaints about government interference in their activities, rarely display any reluctance to benefit from subsidies and taxpayer money.

Americans today spend a smaller percentage of their income on food than any people in the history of the world, and also a smaller amount of time preparing it. We think of that as an achievement and a blessing. But it's not widely recognized that, thanks to misguided farm bills, it's primarily unhealthy foods like feedlot meat, sweetened beverages, and processed foods with added sweeteners and fats that are cheap. The price of fresh fruits and vegetables has been rising steadily for years. It's the food products that are the least healthy that are readily available and inexpensive, because these are the ones that our food policies have been subsidizing rather than healthy foods.

We need to ask what is the real cost of this seemingly cheap fast food. The agricultural systems producing them are destroying rural communities, polluting our water, eroding our topsoil, causing incredible suffering to animals, emitting greenhouse gases at egregious rates, and giving most of us toxic levels of nutritional stress. The CDC estimates that more than one out of every three children born in the U.S. today will develop diabetes as a result of the food they eat. We are paying a terrible price for our seemingly cheap food.

Fast-food companies and other advocates for industrial food production and factory farming say that they are only responding to what people want. Their products are full of sugar and unhealthy fats, they say, because that's what consumers desire. It's not industry's role, they protest, to change people's natural inclinations.

But in fact, the industrial food machine and its allies in government have for many years been at work shaping people's food desires through the way they create food products, package them, sell them, and market them. Companies like Coca-Cola, PepsiCo, Kraft Foods, and McDonald's spend billions of dollars a year marketing junk food to children; they cantankerously fight every effort health advocates make to put any limits whatsoever on their right to target children with ads for fast food, sugary cereals, soft drinks, hot dogs, candy, and other nutrient-deficient products.

In 2011, California Assemblyman Bill Monning proposed legislation that would impose a penny-per-fluid-ounce excise tax on beverages with significant amounts of added sweeteners, like soda pop and sports drinks. The bill would raise $1.7 billion annually that could be used to lower the price of fresh vegetables and fruits for low-income children and families. Not surprisingly, Coca-Cola and PepsiCo aggressively fought the bill. Their representatives castigated the effort as just another attempt by "do-gooders" at "social engineering."

Similar attacks have been leveled against efforts to tax white bread and use the revenue to lower the price of whole-wheat bread, to tax pesticides and use the income to lower the price of organic food, and to tax junk food in order to lower the price of wholesome and nutritious food.

How can we break this cycle? How can we break the cultural trance and overcome the political cowardice that permits industrial fast food and factory farms so much control over both national and state food policies—and ultimately over what most of us eat? How can we obtain foods that are truly nutritious, affordable, and produced in a sustainable way? That, in a nutshell, is the subject of the essays and articles in this book. Each of the pieces in it speaks to steps you can take toward a healthier, more humane, and more Earth-friendly agriculture and cuisine.

No Happy Cows gathers together some of my most widely discussed and circulated blog posts, along with some substantial new writing. These articles cover topics like what's fueling the rise in obesity, whether soy is healthy or harmful, the debate about grass-fed beef, the marketing of junk food to children, why we are seeing a rise in food contamination, the politics and health implications of chocolate and coffee, the perils and broken promises of GMO foods, and hormone disruption in children (and its connection to animal-based foods). There is also a section on the social realities of engaging with people whose food habits are endangering their health.

I hope you enjoy the book, and I hope you find support here for your efforts to live a healthy life. I write from the belief that we can still break through the control that companies like Monsanto have been exerting over our food systems, and bring our agriculture policies back into alignment with the greatest good of our people and the Earth. I write from the conviction that what the Constitution of the United States calls "the general welfare" is more important than the short-term profits of companies whose products are nutritional and environmental disasters.

I write from a faith that it is possible to turn things around. If more Americans stopped overeating, stopped eating unhealthy foods, and instead ate more foods with higher nutrient densities and cancer-protective properties, we could have a more affordable, sustainable, and effective healthcare system. We'd be less dependent on insurance companies and doctors, and more dependent on our own health-giving choices.

We can make healthy choices as individuals, as families, and as a society. We can support farmers' markets, natural food stores, and organic and locally sourced restaurants. We can put restrictions on the right of junk-food companies to bombard children with ads that make them crave foods that are unhealthy for them to eat.

We can stop factory farms from breeding antibiotic-resistant bacteria by prohibiting the indiscriminate use of antibiotics in livestock. We can require factory farms to clean up their own waste, and require them to treat the animals that provide our meat, milk, and eggs with a modicum of decency and respect. It's true that this would raise the price of meat and cause some Americans to eat less, but that would be a good thing not a bad thing. It would improve the health of consumers, livestock, and the land.

If we are going to subsidize any foods, why not make it healthy foods like vegetables, fruits, nuts, and whole grains, rather than high-fructose corn syrup and cattle feeds made from GMO soy and corn? If we are going to subsidize a type of agriculture, why not support family farmers who have a long-term commitment to the land, who are stewards of the Earth, rather than corporate farms that view the land as simply another commodity to be exploited?

Despite the efforts of big agribusinesses, organic produce is already the fastest-growing and most profitable segment of American agriculture, and the number of farmers' markets in the U.S. has more than doubled in the past eight years. Despite the clout of Coca-Cola and PepsiCo, many school districts throughout the country are already banning sodas and junk foods. Despite the belligerence of the livestock industry and farm bureaus, states are increasingly passing referenda on behalf of animal welfare. Despite untold billions being spent promoting fast food and junk food, a large and ever-growing number of people are choosing to eat local, natural, and wholesome foods.

I write to support those of us who are working to build a healthier way of life and a healthier world. I write to support us all in demanding that the companies who produce our food be held accountable for their impact on our Earth, our health, and our future.

You deserve to know the truth about what you eat, where it comes from, and what its impact is on your life and on the world. The more you know, the more power you will have to take effective and meaningful action. The more you know, the better able you will be to bring your food choices into alignment with your purpose and your passion. Your mind will be clearer, your heart will be more at peace, and your body will thank you for the rest of your life.

PART ONE

Caring for All Creatures

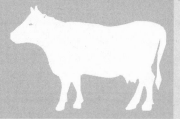

1

The Metamorphosis
of a Pig Farmer

This story, which I first told in The Food Revolution,
*has generated such enthusiastic response that I decided to
include an updated version of it here.*

ONE DAY IN IOWA, I met a particular gentleman—and I
use that term, gentleman, frankly, only because I am trying to be polite, for that is certainly not how I saw him at
the time. He owned and ran what he called a "pork production facility." I, on the other hand, would have called
it a pig Auschwitz.

The conditions were brutal. The pigs were confined in
cages that were barely larger than their own bodies, with
the cages stacked on top of each other in tiers, three high.
The sides and bottoms of the cages were steel slats, so that
excrement from the animals in the upper and middle tiers
dropped through the slats onto the animals below.

The aforementioned owner of this nightmare weighed,
I am sure, at least 240 pounds, but what was even more
impressive about his appearance was that he seemed to be
made out of concrete. His movements had all the fluidity
and grace of a brick wall.

What made him even less appealing was that his language seemed to consist mainly of grunts, many of which sounded alike to me, and none of which were particularly pleasant to hear. Seeing how rigid he was and sensing the overall quality of his presence, I—rather brilliantly, I thought—concluded that his difficulties had not arisen merely because he hadn't had time, that particular morning, to finish his entire daily yoga routine.

But I wasn't about to divulge my opinions of him or his operation, for I was undercover, visiting slaughterhouses and feedlots to learn what I could about modern meat production. There were no bumper stickers on my car, and my clothes and hairstyle were carefully chosen to give no indication that I might have philosophical leanings other than those that were common in the area. I told the farmer matter-of-factly that I was a researcher writing about animal agriculture, and asked if he'd mind speaking with me for a few minutes so that I could have the benefit of his knowledge. In response, he grunted a few words that I could not decipher, but that I gathered meant I could ask him questions and he would show me around.

I was, at this point, not very happy about the situation, and this feeling did not improve when we entered one of the warehouses that housed his pigs. In fact, my distress increased, for I was immediately struck by what I can only call an overpowering olfactory experience. The place reeked in a way you would not believe of ammonia, hydrogen sulfide, and other noxious gases that were the products of the animals' wastes. These, unfortunately, seemed to have been piling up inside the building for far too long.

As nauseating as the stench was for me, I wondered what it must be like for the animals. The cells that detect scent are known as ethmoidal cells. Pigs, like dogs, have nearly 200 times the concentration of these cells in their noses as humans do. In a natural setting, they are able, while rooting around in the dirt, to detect the scent of an edible root through the earth itself.

Given any kind of a chance, pigs will never soil their own nests, for they are actually quite clean animals, despite the reputation we have unfairly given them. But here they had no contact with the earth, and their noses were beset by the unceasing odor of their own urine and feces multiplied 1,000 times by the accumulated wastes of the other pigs unfortunate enough to be caged in that warehouse. I was in the building for only a few minutes, and the longer I remained there, the more desperately I wanted to leave. But the pigs were prisoners there, barely able to take a single step, forced to endure this stench, and almost completely immobile, twenty-four hours a day, seven days a week, and with no time off, I can assure you, for holidays.

The man who ran the place was—I'll give him this—kind enough to answer my questions, which were mainly about the drugs he used to handle the problems that are fairly common in factory pigs today. But my sentiments about him and his farm were not becoming any warmer. It didn't help when, in response to a particularly loud squealing from one of the pigs, he delivered a sudden and threatening kick to the bars of its cage, causing a loud "clang" to reverberate through the warehouse and leading to screaming from many of the pigs.

Because I found it increasingly difficult to hide my distress, it crossed my mind that I should tell the man what I thought of the conditions in which he kept his pigs, but then I thought better of it. This was a man, it was obvious, with whom there was no point in arguing.

After perhaps fifteen minutes, I'd had enough and was preparing to leave. Moreover, I felt sure he was looking forward to getting rid of me. But then something happened, something that changed my life forever—and, as it turns out, his too. It began when his wife came out from the farmhouse and cordially invited me to stay for dinner.

The pig farmer grimaced when his wife spoke, but he dutifully turned to me and announced: "The wife would like you to stay for dinner." He always called her "the wife," by the way, which led me to deduce that he was not, apparently, on the leading edge of feminist thought in the country today.

I don't know whether you have ever done something without having a clue why, and to this day I couldn't tell you what prompted me to do it, but I said "Yes, I'd be delighted." And stay for dinner I did, although I didn't eat the pork they served. The excuse I gave was that my doctor was worried about my cholesterol. I didn't say that I was a vegetarian, or that my cholesterol was 125.

I tried to be a polite and appropriate dinner guest. I didn't want to say anything that might lead to any kind of disagreement. The couple (and their two sons, who were also at the table) were, I could see, being nice to me, giving me dinner and all, and it was gradually becoming clear to me that, along with all the rest of it, they could be, in their way, somewhat decent people. I asked myself whether, if they were traveling in my town and I had chanced to meet them, I would have invited them to dinner. Not likely, I knew—not likely at all. Yet here they were, being as hospitable to me as they could. Yes, I had to admit it. Much as I detested how the pigs were treated, this pig farmer wasn't actually the reincarnation of Adolph Hitler. At least, not at the dinner table.

Of course, I still knew that, if we were to scratch the surface, we'd no doubt find ourselves in great conflict and, because that was not a direction in which I wanted to go, as the meal went along I sought to keep things on an even and consistent keel. Perhaps they sensed it too, for among us, we managed to see that the conversation remained completely and resolutely shallow.

We talked about the weather, about the Little League games in which their two sons played, and then, of course, about how the weather might affect the Little League games. We were actually doing rather well at keeping the conversation superficial and far from any topic around which conflict might occur. Or so I thought. But then suddenly, out of nowhere, the man pointed at me forcefully with his finger, and snarled in a voice that I must say truly frightened me: "Sometimes I wish you animal rights people would just drop dead."

How on Earth he knew I had any affinity to animal rights I will never know—I had painstakingly avoided any mention of any such thing—but I do know that my stomach tightened immediately into a knot. To make matters worse, at that moment his two sons leapt from the table, tore into the den, slammed the door behind them, and turned on the TV, cranking up the volume presumably to drown out what was to follow. At the same instant, his wife nervously picked up some dishes and scurried into the kitchen. As I watched the door close behind her and heard the water begin to run, I had a sinking sensation. They had—there was no mistaking it— left me alone with him.

I was, to put it bluntly, terrified. Under the circumstances, a wrong move now could be disastrous. Trying to center myself, I tried to find some semblance of inner calm by watching my breath, but this I could not do—for the very simple reason that there wasn't any to watch.

"What are they saying that's so upsetting to you?" I said finally, pronouncing the words carefully and distinctly, trying not to show my terror. I was trying very hard at that moment to disassociate myself from the animal rights movement, a force in our society of which he, evidently, was not overly fond.

"They accuse me of mistreating my stock," he growled.

"Why would they say a thing like that?" I answered, knowing full well, of course, why they would, but thinking mostly about my own survival. His reply, to my surprise, while angry, was actually quite articulate. He told me precisely what animal rights groups were saying about operations like his, and exactly why they were opposed to his way of doing things. Then, without pausing, he launched into a tirade about how he didn't like being called cruel, and they didn't know anything about the business he was in, and why couldn't they mind their own business.

As he spoke, the knot in my stomach relaxed, because it was becoming clear—and I was glad of it—that he meant me no harm, but just needed to vent. Part of his frustration, it seemed, was that, even though he didn't like doing some of the things he did to the animals—cooping them up in such small cages, using so many drugs, taking the babies away from their mothers so quickly after their births—he didn't see that he had any choice. He would be at a disadvantage and unable to compete economically if he didn't do things that way. This is how it's done today, he told me, and he had to do it too. He didn't like it, but he liked even less being blamed for doing what he had to do in order to feed his family.

As it happened, I had, just the week before, been at a much larger hog operation, where I learned that it was part of their business strategy to try to put people like my host out of business by going full-tilt into the mass production of assembly-line pigs so that small farmers wouldn't be able to keep up. What I had heard corroborated everything he was saying.

Almost despite myself, I began to grasp the poignancy of this man's human predicament. I was in his home because he and his wife had invited me to be there. And looking around, it was obvious that they were having a hard time making ends meet. Things were threadbare. This family was on the edge.

Raising pigs, apparently, was the only way the farmer knew to make a living, so he did it even though, as was becoming evident the more we talked, he didn't like one bit the direction hog farming was going. At times, as he spoke about how much he hated the modern factory methods of pork production, he reminded me of the very animal rights people who, a few minutes before, he had said he wished would drop dead.

As the conversation progressed, I actually began to develop some sense of respect for this man whom I had earlier judged so harshly. There was decency in him. There was something within him that meant well. But as I began to sense a spirit of goodness in him, I could only wonder all the more how he could treat his pigs the way he did. Little did I know that I was about to find out.

As we talk, he suddenly looks troubled. He slumps over, his head in his hands. He looks broken, and there is a sense of something awful having happened.

Has he had a heart attack? A stroke? I'm finding it hard to breathe, and hard to think clearly. "What's happening?" I ask.

It takes him awhile to answer, but finally he does. I am relieved that he is able to speak, although what he says hardly brings any clarity to the situation. "It doesn't matter," he says, "and I don't want to talk about it." As he speaks, he makes a motion with his hand, as if he were pushing something away.

For the next several minutes, we continue to converse, but I'm quite uneasy. Things seem incomplete and confusing. Something dark has entered the room, and I don't know what it is or how to deal with it.

Then, as we are speaking, it happens again. Once again a look of despondency comes over him. Sitting there, I know I'm in the presence of something bleak and oppressive. I try to be present with what's happening, but it's not easy. Again, I'm finding it hard to breathe.

Finally, he looks at me and I notice his eyes are teary. "You're right," he says. I, of course, always like to be told that I am right, but in this instance, I don't have the slightest idea what he's talking about.

He continues. "No animal," he says, "should be treated like that. Especially hogs. Do you know that they're intelligent animals? They're even friendly, if you treat 'em right. But I don't."

There are tears welling up in his eyes. And he tells me that he has just had a memory come back of something that happened in his childhood, something he hasn't thought of for many years. It's come back in stages, he says.

He grew up, he tells me, on a small farm in rural Missouri, the old-fashioned kind where animals ran around, with barnyards and pastures, and where the animals all had names. I learn, too, that he was an only child, the son of a powerful father who ran things with an iron fist. With no brothers or sisters, he often felt lonely, but found companionship among the animals on the farm, particularly several dogs that were like friends to him. And, he tells me—and this I am quite surprised to hear—he had a pet pig.

As he tells me about this pig, it is as if he becomes a different person. Before, he had spoken primarily in a monotone; now, his voice grows lively. His body language, which until this point seemed to speak primarily of long suffering, now becomes animated. There is something fresh taking place.

In the summer, he tells me, he slept in the barn. It was cooler there than in the house, and the pig often came over to sleep beside him, asking fondly to have her belly rubbed, which he was glad to do.

There was a pond on their property, he goes on, and he liked to swim in it when the weather was hot, but one of the dogs always got excited when he did and ruined things, jumping into the water and swimming up on top of him, scratching him with her paws and making things miserable for him. He was about to give up on swimming, but then, as fate would have it, the pig, of all creatures, stepped in and saved the day.

Evidently the pig could swim, for she plopped herself into the water, swam out to where the dog was bothering him, and inserted herself between them. She stayed between the dog and the boy, keeping the dog at bay. She was, as best I could make out, functioning in the situation something like a lifeguard—or in this case, perhaps more of a life-pig.

As I listen to this hog farmer tell me these stories about his pet pig, I'm thoroughly enjoying both myself and him, and am rather astounded at how things are transpiring. Then, it happens again—a look of defeat sweeps across the man's face and I sense the presence of something very sad. Something in him, I know, is struggling to make its way toward life through anguish and pain, but I don't know what it is or how, indeed, to help him.

"What happened to your pig?" I ask.

He sighs, and it's as if the whole world's pain is contained in that sigh. Then, slowly, he speaks. "My father made me butcher it."

"Did you?" I ask.

"I ran away, but I couldn't hide. They found me."

"What happened?"

"My father gave me a choice."

"What was that?"

"He told me, 'You either slaughter that animal or you're no longer my son.'"

Some choice, I think, feeling the weight of how fathers have so often trained their sons not to care, to be what they call brave and strong, but what so often turns out to be callous and closed-hearted.

"So I did it," he says, and now his tears begin to flow, making their way down his cheeks. I am touched and humbled.

This man, whom I had judged to be without human feeling, is weeping in front of me, a stranger. This man, whom I had seen as callous and even heartless, is actually someone who cares, and deeply. How wrong, how profoundly and terribly wrong, I had been.

In the minutes that follow, it becomes clear to me what has been happening. The pig farmer has remembered something that was so painful, that was such a profound trauma, that he had not been able to cope with it when it happened. Something had shut down then. It was just too much to bear.

Somewhere in his young, formative psyche, he made a resolution never to be that hurt again, never to be that vulnerable again. And he built a wall around the place where the pain had occurred, the place where his love and attachment to that pig was located—his heart. And now here he was, slaughtering pigs for a living—still, I imagined, seeking his father's approval. God, what we men will do, I thought, to get our fathers' acceptance.

I had thought he was a cold and closed human being, but now I saw the truth. His rigidity was not the result of a lack of feeling, as I had thought it was. Quite the opposite: it was a sign of how sensitive he was underneath. For if he had not been so sensitive, he would not have been that hurt, and he would not have needed to put up so massive a wall. The tension in his body that had been so apparent to me upon first meeting him, the body armor that he carried, bespoke how hurt he had been and how much capacity for feeling he carried still, beneath it all.

I had judged him, and had done so, to be honest, mercilessly. But for the rest of the evening I sat with him, humbled and grateful for whatever it was in him that had been strong enough to force this long-buried and deeply painful memory to the surface. And I was glad, too, that I had not stayed stuck in my judgments of him; for if I had, I would not have provided an environment in which his remembering could have occurred.

We talked that night, for hours, about many things. I was, after all that had happened, concerned for him. The gap between his feelings and his lifestyle seemed so tragically vast. What could he do? This was all he knew. He did not have a high school diploma. He was only partially literate. Who would hire him if he tried to do something else? Who would invest in him and train him at his age?

When finally I left that evening, these questions were very much on my mind, and I had no answers to them. Somewhat flippantly, I tried to joke about it. "Maybe," I said, "you'll grow broccoli or something." He stared at me, clearly not comprehending what I could be talking about. It occurred to me, briefly, that possibly he might not know what broccoli was.

We parted that night as friends and, although we rarely saw each other, we remained friends as the years passed. I carry him in my heart and think of him, in fact, as a hero. Because, as you will soon see, impressed as I was by the courage it had taken for him to allow such painful memories to come to the surface, I had not yet seen the extent of his bravery.

When I wrote *Diet for a New America*, I quoted him and summarized what he had told me, but I was quite brief and did not mention his name. I thought that, living as he did among other pig farmers in Iowa, it would not be to his benefit to be associated with me.

When the book came out, I sent him a copy, saying I hoped he was comfortable with how I wrote of the evening we had shared, and directing him to the pages that contained my discussion of our time together.

Several weeks later, I received a letter from him. "Dear Mr. Robbins," it began. "Thank you for the book. When I saw it, I got a migraine headache."

Now, as an author, you do want to have an impact on your readers. This, however, was not what I had had in mind.

He went on, however, to explain that the headaches had gotten so bad that, as he put it, "the wife" suggested that perhaps he should read the book. She thought there might be some kind of connection between the headaches and the book. He told me that this hadn't made much sense to him, but that he had done it because "the wife" was often right about these things.

"You write good," he told me, and I can tell you that these three words of his meant more to me than when the *New York Times* praised the book profusely. He then went on to say that reading the book was very hard for him, because the light it shone on what he was doing made it clear to him that it was wrong to continue. The headaches, meanwhile, kept getting worse. Then that very morning, when he had finished the book after having stayed up all night reading, he went into the bathroom and looked into the mirror. "I decided, right then," he said, "that I would sell my herd and get out of this business. I don't know what I will do, though. Maybe I will, like you said, grow broccoli."

As it happened, he did sell his operation in Iowa and move back to Missouri, where he bought a small farm. He began growing vegetables organically—including, I am sure, broccoli—and selling them at a local farmers' market. He still had pigs, all right, but only about ten of them, and he didn't cage or kill them. Instead, he signed a contract with local schools; they brought children out in buses on field trips to his farm for his "Pet-a-Pig" program. He showed them how intelligent pigs are and how friendly they can be if you treat them right, which he was now doing. He arranged it so that each child got a chance to give a pig a belly rub. He became nearly a vegetarian himself, lost most of his excess weight, and improved his health substantially. And, thank goodness, he actually did better financially than he had been doing before.

He and I corresponded every so often after that. I was very sad to learn, a few years ago, that he had passed away.

Do you see why I still carry this man with me in my heart? Do you see why he is such a hero to me? He dared to leap, to risk everything, to leave what was killing his spirit even though he didn't know what was next. He left behind a way of life that he knew was wrong, and he found one that he knew was right.

When I look at many of the things happening in our world, I sometimes fear we won't make it. But when I remember this man and the power of his spirit, and when I remember that there are many others whose hearts beat to the same quickening pulse, I think we will.

I can get tricked into thinking there aren't enough of us to turn the tide, but then I remember how wrong I was about the pig farmer when I first met him, and I realize that there are heroes everywhere. It's just that I can't recognize them because I think they are supposed to look or act a certain way. How blinded I can be by my own beliefs.

The man is one of my heroes because his example reminds me that we can depart from the cages we build for ourselves and for each other, and become something much better. When I first met him, I would not have thought it possible that I would ever say the things I am saying here. But this only goes to show how amazing life can be, and how you never really know what to expect. This pig farmer has become, for me, a reminder never to underestimate the power of the human heart.

I consider myself privileged to have spent that day with him, and I am grateful that I was allowed to be a catalyst for the unfolding of his spirit. I know my presence served him in some way, but I also know, and know full well, that I received far more than I gave.

To me, this is grace—to have the veils lifted from our eyes so that we can recognize and serve the goodness in each other. Others may wish for great riches, psychic powers, or for ecstatic journeys to mystical planes, but to me, this is the true magic of human life.

2

Eggs and the Chickens
Who Lay Them

EGG LOVERS ARE REJOICING because the USDA, usually the last
to notice anything resembling a genuine nutritional advance,
has announced that eggs are much higher in vitamin D than
previously thought, and also 14 percent lower in cholesterol
than previously believed.

Leaving aside for the moment the question of how it is
that scientific authorities could have been so wrong for so
long about something as basic as the levels of vitamin D and
cholesterol in eggs, the new numbers are happy news indeed
for egg lovers. The egg industry is delighted to report that
you can now eat up to ten eggs a week and still stay under
the recommended limit of 300 mg of cholesterol per day for
healthy adults (provided, of course, that you consume no
other cholesterol at all from any other source).

This is putting a sunny-side-up grin on the faces of those
who enjoy eating eggs and don't fancy eating their way to a
heart attack. But if it's enough to make egg lovers smile, it's
like mainlining Prozac for the egg industry—which, as you
might expect, is wasting no time trumpeting the news that
their products have been exonerated.

But wait a minute. There's something that's being over-
looked in all the hoopla—something that may be even more

important than the milligrams of cholesterol in an egg. Do we care how the hens are treated? Do we care about the conditions in which they live and the quality of the food they are fed? Do we care if the eggs are produced humanely and sustainably? If the new dietary information means we'll be eating more eggs that come from sick hens that live in abject misery, is that such a good thing?

The sad fact of modern industrialized egg production is that layer hens are crammed together in filthy cages so small that the birds are not able to lift a wing. The amount of space the birds are given is less than they would have if you stuffed several of them into a file drawer. One building frequently houses 30,000 hens packed together.

The birds are driven so insane by these miserable conditions that they would peck each other to death if they could. The industry, of course, doesn't want to see such a thing happen, because there's no profit to be made from dead hens who don't lay eggs. How, then, does the industry prevent it? Not by giving the hens more room, which would be the humane response. Instead, they cut off a sizable part of the hens' beaks—a process known euphemistically as "beak trimming."

What's a concerned consumer to do? Fortunately, the Cornucopia Institute has come out with an Organic Egg Scorecard that empowers consumers with accurate information. The scorecard rates companies that sell name-brand and private-label organic eggs against the criteria that are most important to the majority of conscientious consumers.

There are two things the Organic Egg Scorecard quickly makes apparent.

The first is that just because eggs are "organic" doesn't mean they are humanely raised. In fact, there are "organic" factory-farm operations with more than 80,000 "organic" hens in a single building.

The second thing the Organic Egg Scorecard reveals is exactly which brands of eggs found in your local stores are produced using the best organic practices and with the most ethical regard for the hens. If you are interested in which eggs are sustainable and humane and which are not, check it out.

The results may surprise you. For example, the private label brands sold by Trader Joe's, Safeway OOrganics, Walmart's Great Value, and Costco's Kirkland Signature get the lowest possible rating because these companies were unable or unwilling to provide any meaningful information about how their chickens are housed, fed, or treated. Unfortunately, the Cornucopia Institute reports, "the vast majority of organic eggs for private label brands are produced on industrial farms that house hundreds of thousands of birds and do not grant the birds meaningful outdoor access."

Many egg suppliers tout that their eggs are produced without hormones. That sounds great but is, in fact, meaningless because, unlike beef and dairy products, no eggs produced in the U.S. today are legally produced with hormones. Federal regulations prohibit the use of hormones in raising poultry.

Whole Foods, at least, has taken a step in the right direction by not selling any eggs that come from hens whose beaks have been "trimmed." Whole Foods shoppers can take some comfort in knowing that eggs bought there do not come from the worst of the nation's egg factories.

If you want to consume eggs from healthy and happy hens, you may want to take a step in the direction of food self-reliance and keep a few hens in your backyard. Or get your eggs from a neighbor or from a small-scale farm you can actually visit. Or purchase only eggs that are highly rated by the Organic Egg Scorecard.

Personally, my favorite breakfast is guaranteed to be cruelty-free. It's oatmeal with cinnamon, raisins, and walnuts, which aren't added only for flavor. Oats are a comparatively low-glycemic-index grain to begin with, but the addition of walnuts creates a nourishing breakfast with high protein content, high nutrient density, a healthy form of fat, and a very low glycemic index.

Here's my recipe for a tasty and hearty breakfast that will provide you with consistent blood sugar levels, and give you plenty of energy all morning. Serves three.

1 cup rolled oats
3 cups water
½ teaspoon salt
½ teaspoon cinnamon
⅓ cup raisins
⅓ cup walnuts

1. Place oats, water, salt, cinnamon, and raisins in a covered saucepan and bring to a boil.

2. Turn down heat and simmer for 10 minutes, stirring occasionally.

3. Remove from heat, stir in walnuts, and serve hot.

3

No Such Thing as Happy Cows

As THE ONLY SON OF THE FOUNDER of the Baskin-Robbins ice cream empire, I grew up eating plenty of ice cream and being groomed to take over the family business. It was painful for me to face the fact that the sale and consumption of ice cream was contributing to rising rates of heart disease and obesity. And it was even more painful to learn that ice cream was made from milk that was produced at the cost of tremendous suffering for the dairy cows and their calves. Instead of following in my father's footsteps, I turned away from the family business and committed myself to working for a more compassionate and healthy world.

In my books, including *Diet for a New America* and *The Food Revolution*, I detail the horrific abuses suffered by animals like dairy cows and their calves in large-scale animal operations. These books have become international bestsellers, which has reinforced my belief that these are issues of importance to an increasing number of people.

In 2010, California Governor Arnold Schwarzenegger signed a bill that prohibits any egg from being sold in the state that comes from caged hens; the bill takes effect in 2015. This bill became law twenty months after a 63 percent majority of California voters approved Proposition 2, the Prevention of Farm Animal Cruelty Act, which made it clear that concern for the living conditions of livestock is no longer the province of animal rights activists alone.

Recognizing that concern about the humane treatment of farm animals has been growing, the California Milk Advisory Board proceeded to ramp up its ten-year "Happy Cow" advertising campaign with a new series of ads proclaiming: "Great milk comes from Happy Cows. Happy Cows come from California." These ads are now being shown across the nation.

Unfortunately, there are a few problems with the ads. For one, they aren't always 100 percent loyal to the truth. As an example, they weren't filmed in California at all. They were filmed in Auckland, New Zealand.

Unfortunately, that's just the tip of the iceberg.

The California Milk Board has suffused the state with billboards and other ads proudly proclaiming that 99 percent of the state's dairy farms are family owned. But in order to arrive at this figure, they include each and every rural household in the state that happens to have one or two cows, and calls each of them a dairy farm. In this calculation, each of these households is counted as a single dairy farm and given the same weight as a corporate-owned dairy in the San Joaquin Valley that has 20,000 cows. Consumers reading the billboards and other ads may think that most of the state's milk comes from family farms when, in fact, 95 percent of the milk produced in the state comes from large corporate dairies.

Thanks to the practices these corporate dairies employ, the amount of milk produced yearly by the average California cow is nearly 3,000 pounds more than the national average. This increased production may seem like a good thing, but it is achieved at great cost to the animals. The cows are routinely confined in extremely unnatural conditions, injected with hormones, fed antibiotics, and in general treated without compassion like four-legged milk pumps. The ads portray California's cows as happy when, in actuality, one third of California's cows suffer from painful udder infections, and more than half suffer from other infections and illnesses.

The natural lifespan of a dairy cow is about twenty years, but California's dairy cows are typically slaughtered when they are four or five years old, because they've become crippled from painful foot infections or calcium depletion, or simply because they can no longer produce the unnaturally high amounts of milk required of them.

It's hard to see how the life of the average California cow today could legitimately be considered to be a happy one, which raises a few questions. Are we going to hold our advertisers accountable to reality? Are we going to ask that what they tell us bears some resemblance to the truth? The California Milk Advisory Board has built an advertising campaign that portrays the life of these animals as one of ease and comfort. The Milk Board is pleased with the Happy Cow ads, and is pouring hundreds of millions of dollars into presenting them to the nation. But is this ad campaign deceiving consumers?

The ads—with slogans like "So much grass, so little time"— present the California dairy industry as a bucolic enterprise that operates in lush, grassy pastures that look remarkably like, well, New Zealand. It sounds nice, except for the fact that California's dairy industry is concentrated in the dry and barren Central Valley. Here, the cows are typically kept in overcrowded dirt feedlots. Some never see a blade of grass in their entire lives.

Perhaps a more accurate slogan would be: "So many cows, so little space."

The ads show calves in meadows talking happily to their mothers. But the reality is a little different. Male calves born to California dairy cows typically spend only twenty-four hours with their mothers, and some do not even get that much. They are then taken from their mothers to be slaughtered, or condemned to languish tethered within the small confines of veal crates.

The ads happily give the impression that the practices of the dairy industry are in harmony with the environment. But once again, this lovely picture isn't entirely accurate. The 1,600 dairies in California's Central Valley produce more excrement than the entire human population of Texas. The amount of waste produced each year by the dairy cows in the fifty-square-mile area of California's Chino Basin would make a pile with the dimensions of a football field and as tall as the Empire State Building. When it rains heavily, dairy manure in the Chino Basin is washed straight into the Santa Ana River. A considerable amount of it inevitably makes its way into the aquifer that supplies half of Orange County's drinking water.

One thing the Happy Cow ads never mention is that 20 million Californians (65 percent of the state's population) rely on drinking water that is threatened by contamination from nitrates and other poisons stemming from dairy manure. Nitrates have been linked to cancer and birth defects.

It's been said that "ignorance is bliss," and it may be that a certain level of happiness is possible when we don't look too closely at things that make us uncomfortable. The Milk Board, which seems to thrive on our ignorance, never gets around to mentioning that genetically engineered bovine growth hormone is widely used in California's largest dairy operations to increase milk production. Nor that the hormone is banned in many countries—including Canada, Australia, New Zealand, and much of the European Union—because it increases udder infections and lameness in the cows, markedly raises the amount of pus found in milk, and may increase the risk of cancer in consumers.

Many consumers today are willing to pay extra for products that have been produced humanely and with respect for the environment. If someone produces eggs from free-range chickens, they can get a higher price in the marketplace than they could for conventionally produced eggs. If someone makes bread made from organically grown wheat, they can get a higher price for it. But what if someone were to tell the public that their eggs were free-range when this was false, or were to tell the public that the wheat in their bread was organic when this wasn't true? Would their actions be considered dishonest? Would they be seen as attempting to take unfair advantage of the public? Might their dishonesty even be considered criminal? Why, then, do we allow the Milk Board's Happy Cow ad campaign to portray California dairy products as humanely produced in harmony with the environment? Why do we allow them to take advantage of the people who care enough about this precious Earth and the life it holds to pay a higher price for foods produced with respect for life?

The Milk Board defends the ads by saying they are entertaining, and are not intended to be taken seriously. However, the Milk Board does not appear to me to be in the entertainment business. Is it spending hundreds of millions of dollars on this ad campaign to amuse the public, or to increase the sales of California dairy products?

The Milk Board says the ads show talking cows, and no one thinks cows talk. Therefore, they conclude, the ads are not misleading. They are right, of course, that no one in their right mind thinks cows talk. And they are right that their ads do not mislead people into believing they do. But I am not aware of a movement of consumers demanding animal products from talking animals. There are, however, a large number of consumers who care about animals and the planet, and who are willing to pay extra for humanely raised animal products and products raised in Earth-friendly ways.

The Milk Board knows that showing calves being ripped away from their mothers and confined in tiny veal crates won't sell their product. Neither will showing emaciated, lame animals that have collapsed from a lifetime of hardship and over-milking being taken to slaughterhouses and having their throats slit. But this is the sad reality of the California dairy industry. Covering up this misery with fantasy ads of happy cows does nothing to alleviate the suffering these animals endure.

This is why I have joined with People for the Ethical Treatment of Animals (PETA) in a lawsuit that challenges the Milk Board's ads as unlawfully deceptive. To my eyes, it is inhumane to inflict widespread suffering on cows and their calves. I consider it inexcusable to poison the state's groundwater basins. And I think it is dishonest to deceive caring consumers about this animal suffering and environmental devastation. Thus I would feel irresponsible if I sat by and did nothing while the Milk Board continues to spend hundreds of millions of dollars on their Happy Cow ad campaign.

After joining the lawsuit, I was interviewed by a skeptical reporter, who asked some provocative questions about my participation. A portion of our dialogue follows:

Question: Don't you think the ads are funny?

Answer: I think they are clever, but as someone who takes animal suffering seriously, I don't find them humorous. There's nothing funny about cruelty, and I don't think that misleading the public becomes legitimate when it is done in an "entertaining" way.

Question: You are joined in this lawsuit by PETA. Aren't your complaints about the ads something that only animal rights advocates would make?

Answer: Consumers who want the animal products they buy to be from humanely raised animals can be found in every segment of society. McDonald's has recently increased the size of the cages in which their chickens are kept, and decreased the number of birds in the cages. They have made this change at considerable cost, because they recognize the strength of the market demand from their customer base for more humanely raised poultry. Burger King and Taco Bell have made similar changes. The customer bases for these fast-food franchises are not made up of animal rights advocates. On the contrary, they are composed of mainstream Americans. Consideration for the plight of animals is a central part of the American character. It is an essential part of who we are as a people. Abraham Lincoln was not speaking only for animal rights advocates when he said: "I care not much for a man's religion whose dog or cat aren't the better for it." I think the Happy Cow ads are an insult to the legitimate humanitarian concerns of millions of people.

Question: Are you joining this lawsuit because you are a vegetarian?

Answer: No. Being a vegetarian is a personal choice. It is not a personal choice whether you tell the truth about products you are marketing to the public. In fact, it is the non-vegetarian population that is more the victim of this ad campaign. Many vegetarians do not consume any kind of dairy products, so this kind of false advertising actually affects them less.

Question: Aren't all ads like this? When I buy a beer, I don't expect to get two women in bikinis standing next to me.

Answer: It's true that many ads exploit the desires of people for happier and more exciting lives. But to me, the Happy Cow campaign seems uniquely irresponsible. Our society is not experiencing a concerted and serious social movement composed of people from all walks of life demanding that commercial beer products come with women in bikinis. There is, however, exactly that kind of movement demanding that dairy and other animal food products come from humanely treated animals and environmentally sustainable practices.

Question: The ads imply that California cows are treated better than cows in other states. Is this true?

Answer: No. The reality is actually the opposite. California's dairy industry is concentrated for the most part in the dry

Central Valley, which is now the number one milk-producing area in the United States. Here, the cows are typically kept in dirt feedlots, unlike the green pastoral fields common in Wisconsin, for example, where there is much higher annual rainfall. California dairy cows are kept in larger numbers in smaller areas than anywhere else in the country.

Question: What are you trying to accomplish with this lawsuit?

Answer: We are asking the court to take animal suffering seriously, and to put a stop to these deceptive ads. Furthermore, I would like to see the dairy industry make amends and make an effort to rectify some of the damage done by the ads. For example, I would like to see the Milk Board pay fines at a level commensurate with what they've paid for the Happy Cow campaign. And I'd like to see that money used to fund a public service educational campaign to educate people of all ages about the importance of preventing cruelty to animals.

Question: What is the current status of the lawsuit?

Answer: Thus far, the Milk Board has prevailed in court. Why? Because the California Milk Advisory Board is the marketing arm of the California Department of Agriculture, which is a government agency. And in California, in a truly Orwellian twist, government agencies are exempt from laws prohibiting false advertising.

Question: If the courts won't step in and protect us, what can we do?

Answer: I think it's time for consumers to stop rewarding this behavior with our hard-earned dollars. I think it's time for us to withdraw our support from industries that mislead us and whose practices are cruel to animals. I think it's time for us to understand that, when it comes to factory farms, there are no happy cows.

PART TWO

What Are We Putting into Our Bodies?

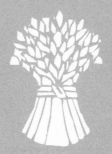

4

Health Food or Harm Food? The Truth about Soy

IN RECENT YEARS, I've received quite a number of requests from people asking for my views on soy products. Many of these inquiries have mentioned a stridently anti-soy article written by Sally Fallon and Mary G. Enig titled "Tragedy and Hype" that has been widely circulated. This article presents a systematic series of accusations against soy consumption, and has formed the basis for many similar articles. Many people, as a result, are now seriously questioning the safety of soy.

The litany of dangers of soy products, according to Fallon and Enig, is nearly endless. Tofu, they say, shrinks brains and causes Alzheimer's. Soy products promote rather than prevent cancer. Soy contains "anti-nutrients" and is full of toxins. The pro-soy publicity of the past few years is nothing but "propaganda." Soy formula, they say, amounts to "birth control pills for babies."

"Soy is not hemlock," they conclude; "Soy is more insidious than hemlock."

Fallon and Enig say the soy industry knows soy is poisonous, and "lie(s) to the public to sell more soy." They say that soy is "the next asbestos." They predict that there will be huge lawsuits with "thousands and thousands of legal briefs." They warn that those who will be held legally responsible for deliberately manipulating the public to make money "include merchants, manufacturers, scientists, publicists, bureaucrats, former bond financiers, food writers, vitamin companies, and retail stores."

Given the rapidly expanding role that soy in its many forms has come to play in the Western diet, these accusations are extremely serious. If they are true, the widespread trust that many people have come to have in soy is not only misplaced, but disastrous.

Soy foods have come to play such a significant role in the diets of many health-conscious people, and the allegations that have been made against them are so many and so grave, that I think the topic warrants a careful, detailed, and meticulous look. What follows is my attempt to provide an objective appraisal of both the benefits and the dangers of soy.

BLESSING OR CURSE?

Not that long ago, soybeans were considered by most Americans to be "hippie food." But then medical research began accumulating that affirmed that soy consumption reduced heart disease and cancer risk, that it lengthened life and enhanced its quality, and that it provided an almost ideal protein substitute for animal proteins that almost inevitably come packaged with cholesterol and unhealthy forms of saturated fat. The mainstream culture began taking note. In a 1999 article titled "The Joy of Soy," *Time Magazine* announced that consuming a mere 1.5 ounces of soy a day can significantly lower both total and LDL ("bad") cholesterol levels. The evidence was becoming so convincing that even the ardently pro-pharmaceutical FDA wound up affirming that soybeans are a food that can prevent and even cure disease.

As the evidence of soy's health benefits accumulated, sales and consumption skyrocketed. Books like *The Simple Soybean and Your Health, Tofu Cookery,* and *The Book of Tofu* helped spread the word. Annual soy milk sales, which amounted to only a few million dollars in the early 1980s, have now soared to more than a billion dollars. And it's not just soy milk; it's all soy foods. From 1996 to 2011, annual soy food sales in the U.S. literally quintupled—increasing from $1 billion to $5 billion.

But, according to Fallon and Enig, this is all a tragic mistake, because soy is far indeed from living up to the many health claims that its proponents have made for it. Quite the contrary, they say: "[T]he soybean contains large quantities of natural toxins or 'antinutrients,' (including) potent enzyme inhibitors that block the action of trypsin and other enzymes needed for protein digestion. . . . They can produce serious distress, reduced protein digestion, and chronic deficiencies in amino acid uptake."

These are serious allegations, because soy is often consumed precisely for its considerable protein levels. In my view, there is a kernel of truth behind these charges, though one that Fallon and Enig greatly overstate. It is true that the protein in cooked soybeans is slightly less digestible than that found in most animal foods. However, when soybeans are made into soy milk, tofu, tempeh, and the other common forms of soy foods, their protein digestibility is enhanced and becomes similar to animal foods. Any negative impact on protein digestibility due to the presence of the enzyme inhibitors found in soybeans is rendered nearly irrelevant in these foods. And even simple soybeans, with their reduced digestibility, are so high in protein and in all the essential amino acids that they could still easily serve as the sole source of protein in a person's diet if that were necessary for some reason.

"Soybeans also contain haemagglutinin," continue Fallon and Enig, "a clot-promoting substance that causes red blood cells to clump together. Trypsin inhibitors and haemagglutinin are growth inhibitors. . . . Soy also contains goitrogens—substances that depress thyroid function." It is true that soybeans contain these substances. How then do we explain that moderate amounts of soy foods have been eaten happily by entire civilizations for thousands of years? Fallon and Enig's case is built on animal studies in which test animals fed extremely large and unnatural amounts of soy containing these substances "failed to grow normally" and developed "pathological conditions of the pancreas, including cancer." But the fact is that there is little or no evidence that the quantities of these substances found in a typical diet including soybeans represents a health danger to humans.

ANIMAL STUDIES

Animal studies are at the very foundation of many of the accusations against soy. But humans are different from any other animal, so foods that affect them in one way may well affect us differently. Protease inhibitors are substances that retard the action of digestive enzymes that cause the breakdown of protein. Fallon and Enig refer to studies that show that protease inhibitors isolated from soybeans can cause cancer in some animal species, but there is no evidence even suggesting that they have the same effect in humans. In fact, protease inhibitors found in soybeans have been shown to reduce the incidence of colon, prostate, and breast cancer in humans.

Fallon and Enig make much of a 1985 study that showed that soy increases the risk of pancreatic cancer in rats. But researchers with the National Cancer Institute point out that the pancreas of a few species of animals—notably rats and chicks—are extraordinarily sensitive to dietary protease inhibitors like those found in soy. This sensitivity has not been found in other species like hamsters, mice, dogs, pigs, and monkeys, they say, and is "not expected to occur in humans." In fact, while rats fed nothing but soy run higher risks of pancreatic cancer, human populations consuming high levels of soy have decreased rates of pancreatic cancer.

Species, even those that seem quite closely related, often function quite differently at a molecular level. It is true, as Fallon and Enig point out, that baby rats fail to thrive on soy. But they also fail to thrive on human breast milk. This is because rats and humans have vastly different nutritional requirements. Human milk, for example, is 5 percent protein; rats' milk is 45 percent protein. The difference in nutritional requirements and responses for different species can be enormous. Foods that are highly nutritious for one species are often inedible or even poisonous to other species.

Soybeans are high in isoflavones—phytoestrogens, or plant substances that behave like weak forms of the hormone estrogen. Fallon and Enig select a few animal studies that appear to show a correlation between soy isoflavone consumption and cancer risk. But soy consumption has been found repeatedly to *lower* breast cancer risk in humans, precisely because of the isoflavones in it.

Why the difference? Dr. K. O. Kline of the Department of Clinical Science at DuPont Hospital for Children in Delaware, comments in a 1998 article in *Nutrition Reviews*. "It is clear from the literature," writes Kline, "that different species and different tissues are affected by (soy) isoflavones in markedly different ways." Fallon and Enig, however, do not agree. They denounce Kline's comments, fuming that "this is scientific double talk." Another interpretation may be that Kline is simply acknowledging the reality that there are physiological differences between species that must be taken into account.

Remember thalidomide, the drug that caused horrendous birth defects in children born to mothers who took the drug during their pregnancies? Thalidomide had been widely tested on animals, where it appeared to be totally safe. Similarly, the combination of fenfluramine and dexfenfluramine, recently touted to be the answer to dieters' prayers, was extensively tested on animals and found to be very safe. Unfortunately it caused heart-valve abnormalities in humans. When the arthritis drug Opren was tested on monkeys, no problems were found, but it killed sixty-one people before it was withdrawn. Cylert was fine for animals, but when it was given to hyperactive children it caused liver failure.

THE CANCER CONNECTION

The important question, then, is what is the relationship between soy consumption and cancer in humans? Despite the allegations of those wishing to build a case against soy, the evidence strongly suggests not only that soy does not promote cancer; it reduces cancer risk.

For example, the elders of Okinawa have repeatedly been shown to be the healthiest and longest-lived people in the world. This was demonstrated conclusively in the renowned Okinawa Centenarian Study, a twenty-five-year study sponsored by the Japanese Ministry of Health.

The researchers conducting the study analyzed the diet and health profiles of Okinawan elders, and compared them with other elder populations throughout the world. They concluded that high soy consumption is one of the main reasons that Okinawans are at extremely low risk for hormone-dependent cancers, including cancers of the breast, prostate, ovaries, and colon. Compared with North Americans, they have a staggering 80 percent less breast and prostate cancer, and less than half the ovarian and colon cancers.

This enormously reduced cancer risk arises in part, the study's authors say, from the Okinawans large consumption of isoflavones from soy. This is an important finding. The lowest cancer rates in the world are found in the Okinawans who consume the most soy.

Other studies have confirmed the link between soy consumption and reduced cancer risk. The Japan Public Health Center Study found the lowest breast cancer rates in prefectures where women ate the most soy products. A recent study published in the British medical journal *Lancet* showed that women who ate the most flavonoids (mostly isoflavones from soy products) had a substantially lower risk of breast cancer than those who had lower flavonoid intake.

Perhaps most telling, a huge study published in *The Journal of the National Cancer Institute* in 2003 found that women with a high intake of soy reduced their risk of breast cancer by 54 percent compared with women with a low intake of soy.

The anti-soy campaigners repeatedly say that soy foods raise the risk of cancer. But such charges are utterly incompatible with the findings of the prestigious Health Professionals Follow-up Study, which found a 70 percent reduction in prostate cancer among men who consume soy milk daily.

Kaayla Daniel is a protégé of Fallon and Enig and the author of a prominent anti-soy book, *The Whole Soy Story: The Dark Side of America's Favorite Health Food*. The book is edited by Fallon, who owns the small book company that publishes it. In her book, Daniel says that "soy can almost certainly be blamed for at least some of the increase in thyroid cancers in that soy isoflavones [the type of phytoestrogen found in soy] induce . . . thyroid tumors." But that's not what the Cancer Prevention Institute of California found when it undertook the Bay Area Thyroid Cancer Study. Quite the contrary. They found that those who consumed the most phytoestrogens from soy foods, whole grains, nuts, and seeds had a markedly lower risk of thyroid cancer. Women who consumed the most soy had about half the risk of thyroid cancer compared with those who consumed the least.

It is true that if you eat too much soy and your diet is deficient in iodine, your thyroid gland may become swollen and underactive, you may develop symptoms of hypothyroidism (such as lethargy and depression), and your risk of thyroid cancer could increase. But the answer isn't to avoid soy. It's to make sure you consume enough iodine. Soy does not cause thyroid problems in people who consume adequate amounts of iodine.

In the U.S., iodine deficiency is very rare because common table salt is fortified with it, and a mere quarter teaspoon of iodized salt provides the needed daily dose. Those not consuming iodized salt, however, should make sure they are obtaining reliable sources of the mineral. The iodine content of plant foods depends greatly on the amounts found in the soil in which they are grown. Sea vegetables and seaweeds are excellent and reliable sources of the mineral, and most multivitamin supplements contain iodine.

Meanwhile, Kaayla Daniel's book has misled many health-conscious people into believing that soy increases the risk not only for thyroid problems and thyroid cancer, but for many other forms of cancer. As a result, an increasing number of people have become frightened of eating soy.

Health researcher Syd Baumel was one of the first to challenge the promotion of soy as a miracle food, and to question the idea that the more soy you eat the better. But when he looked into Daniel's claims, he was anything but impressed. He says Daniel's book "consistently deceives and manipulates the reader in order to build a false case. . . . Pretty well anywhere you dip into this book, the waters are muddied with half-truths, misrepresentations, errors, lies and other tricks of false persuasion." Baumel gives this example:

> Daniel cites a five-year clinical trial in which six out of
> 179 post-menopausal women taking a very high dosage soy isoflavone supplement developed endometrial

hyperplasia. None of the 197 women who took a placebo did. "Endometrial proliferation is a precursor of cancer," Daniel warns, implying the women can look forward to a date with the oncologist. She doesn't mention that all of them developed the relatively benign, non-atypical form of endometrial hyperplasia. Research suggests this condition carries a 2 percent risk of progressing to endometrial cancer—little different from the 1 to 2 percent risk for women in general.

In 1997, the American Institute for Cancer Research, in collaboration with its international affiliate the World Cancer Research Fund, issued a major international report—"Food, Nutrition and the Prevention of Cancer: A Global Perspective." This report analyzed more than 4,500 research studies, and its production involved the participation of more than 120 contributors and peer reviewers, including participants from the World Health Organization, the Food and Agriculture Organization of the United Nations, the International Agency on Research in Cancer, and the U.S. National Cancer Institute. In 2000, Riva Bitrum, President of Research for the American Institute for Cancer Research, said, "Studies showing consistently that just one serving a day of soy foods contributes to a reduction in cancer risk are encouraging."

Of course, any foods with such potent biological properties—even healthful ones—are bound to have some unwanted side effects in some people under some circumstances. Although soy consumption on the whole reduces cancer incidence, there are questions about its effect on women who have estrogen-positive (ER+) breast tumors. These tumors are stimulated by estrogen. Could they therefore be stimulated by the weak estrogenic activity of the isoflavones found in soy? The jury is still out. There is some evidence this may be the case, although there is also evidence that soy consumption favorably alters the metabolism of estrogen so that it is less likely to stimulate tumor growth. For healthy women, according to the American Institute for Cancer Research, "even two or three servings a day of soy foods should be fine as one part of a mostly plant-based diet."

Soy supplements are a different story. Soy pills and powders can contain amounts of isoflavones (usually daidzein and genistein) far in excess of the amounts available through diet. Very little research has been done on the effects of such mega-doses. Although there is no firm evidence to demonstrate that ingestion of isoflavones has adverse effects on human beings, there is also no clear evidence that large doses are safe. Some manufacturers of soy-protein isolates and supplements recommend that people consume 100 grams of soy protein a day (the equivalent of seven or eight soy burgers). I believe it's probably safer, until more is learned, to avoid concentrated soy supplements entirely.

SOY AND MINERAL ABSORPTION

Fallon and Enig are adamant in their beef with soy, however, and their indictment of the bean continues. They fault soy for its phytic acid content. "Soybeans are high in phytic acid," they say, "a substance that can block the uptake of essential minerals—calcium, magnesium, copper, iron, and especially zinc in the intestinal tract. . . . Vegetarians who consume tofu as a substitute for meat and dairy products risk severe mineral deficiencies."

It is true that soybeans are high in phytates, as are many other plant foods like other beans, grains, nuts, and seeds. And it is true that phytates can block the uptake of essential minerals, particularly zinc. This may be a problem if a person consumes enormous amounts of soy. But the phytic acid levels found in a plant-strong diet including as many as three servings of soy a day are not high enough to cause mineral absorption problems for most people. Furthermore, when soy products are fermented—as they are in tempeh, miso, and many other soy foods—phytate levels are reduced to about a third of their initial level. Other methods of soy preparation such as soaking, roasting, and sprouting also significantly reduce phytate content.

While phytates can compromise mineral absorption to some degree, there is absolutely no reliable evidence that vegetarians who eat soy foods "risk severe mineral deficiencies." Even the National Cattlemen's Beef Association has acknowledged the nutritional adequacy of meatless diets. In an official statement, these representatives of the beef industry declared: "Well planned vegetarian diets can meet dietary recommendations for essential nutrients."

Let's look, one by one, at the minerals Fallon and Enig claim to be lacking for those who consume tofu rather than meat:

Zinc: It is wise for vegetarians to include plenty of zinc-rich foods in their diets, but the levels of zinc found in the hair, saliva, and blood of vegetarians are typically in the normal range. Zinc deficiency can be particularly harmful in pregnant women, but studies of pregnant women have consistently found no difference in zinc levels between vegetarians and non-vegetarians.

Iron: Plant-strong diets are much higher in vitamin C, and vitamin C greatly enhances iron absorption. So even without eating red meat (which is high in iron), and even with the reduction in iron absorption from phytates, vegetarians are no more prone to iron deficiency than are non-vegetarians.

Copper: Vegetarian diets tend to be higher in copper, which overrides any reduced rate of absorption from phytates.

Vegans, in particular, consume considerably more copper than meat-eaters.

Magnesium: Although the higher phytate content of soybeans and grains slightly reduces magnesium absorption, vegetarian diets are typically so much higher in this crucial mineral that vegetarians consistently show markedly higher serum magnesium levels than do non-vegetarians.

Calcium: Calcium from soy is nearly as bio-available as calcium from cow's milk. Many studies have found a correlation between the consumption of isoflavones from soy foods and increased bone health.

SOY FOODS AND BONE HEALTH

Without providing any supporting evidence, Fallon and Enig go on to say that "soyfoods block calcium and cause vitamin D deficiencies. . . . The reason that Westerners have such high rates of osteoporosis is because they have substituted soy oil for butter, which is a traditional source of vitamin D . . . needed for calcium absorption."

Vitamin D is indeed needed for calcium absorption, and is crucial to human health in many other ways. But skin exposure to sunlight, not butter consumption, has always been the primary source of vitamin D in humans. In fact, people whose skin is not exposed to direct sunlight have difficulty getting enough vitamin D from their diets without supplementation. A 1999 report in *The American Journal of Clinical Nutrition* said that blood levels of vitamin D in sunlight-deficient people don't begin to rise until 4,000 units of vitamin D are consumed. Someone relying on unfortified butter for this amount would have to eat four pounds of butter a day.

Why, then, do Westerners have such high rates of osteoporosis? We have become sedentary, and we consume a highly processed, high-salt, high-animal-protein diet.

The calcium-draining effect of animal protein on the human body is not a matter of controversy in scientific circles. Researchers who conducted a recent survey of diet and hip fractures in thirty-three countries said they found "an absolutely phenomenal correlation" between the percentage of plant foods in people's diets and the strength of their bones. The more plant foods people eat (particularly fruits and vegetables), the stronger their bones, and the fewer fractures they experience. The more animal foods people eat, on the other hand, the weaker their bones and the more fractures they experience.

Similarly, in January 2001, *The American Journal of Clinical Nutrition* published a study that reported a dramatic correlation between the ratio of animal to vegetable protein in the diets of elderly women and their rate of bone loss. In this seven-year study funded by the National Institutes of Health, more than 1,000 women ages sixty-five to eighty were grouped into three categories: those with a high ratio of animal to vegetable protein, those who fell into a middle range, and those who fell into a low range. The women in the high-ratio category had three times the rate of bone loss as the women in the low-ratio group, and nearly four times the rate of hip fractures.

Could this have been due to other factors than the ratio of animal to vegetable protein? According to the study's lead author, Dr. Deborah Sellmeyer, Director of the Bone Density Clinic at the University of California San Francisco Medical Center, researchers found this to be true even after adjusting for age, weight, estrogen use, tobacco use, exercise, calcium intake, and total protein intake. "We adjusted for all the things that could have had an impact on the relationship of high animal protein intake to bone loss and hip fractures," Sellmeyer said. "But we found the relationship was still there."

SOY AND HEART DISEASE

If the articles written and spawned by Fallon and Enig are credible, just about everything we've been taught to believe about soy's benefits is completely backward. What about soy's vaunted reputation (and FDA approval) for bringing down cholesterol levels? "For most of us," say Fallon and Enig, "giving up steak and eating veggie burgers instead will not bring down blood cholesterol levels."

Someone once said that people are entitled to their own opinions, but not to their own facts. A review of thirty-eight studies published in *The New England Journal of Medicine* in 1995 found that soy consumption reduced cholesterol levels in 89 percent of the studies.

If there is a grain of truth in Fallon and Enig's statement, it is that while soy consumption tends to bring down total cholesterol levels most in people whose cholesterol levels are high, the results are less dramatic in those with healthier levels. But even people with normal levels benefit from eating more soy, according to dozens of studies, because it improves the ratio between HDL (good) and LDL (bad) cholesterol. This ratio is now recognized by the American Heart Association to be an even more important factor than total cholesterol levels in heart-disease risk.

In 2000, the Nutrition Committee of the American Heart Association published a major statement in the peer-reviewed journal *Circulation*, officially recommending the inclusion of 25 grams or more of soy protein, with its associated phytochemicals intact (i.e., not in the form of an isolated soy-protein supplement), in the daily diet as a means of promoting heart health. This recommendation is consistent with the FDA's ruling allowing soy protein products to carry the health claim: "25 grams/day of soy protein, as part of a diet low in saturated fat and cholesterol, may reduce the risk of heart disease."

What do the soy pooh-pooh-ers say to this? They say that lowered cholesterol levels, even those lowered by diet, are dangerous: "The truth is that cholesterol is your best friend," they write. "When cholesterol levels in the blood are high, it's because the body needs cholesterol. . . . There is no greater risk of heart disease at cholesterol levels of 300 than at 180."

That's quite a point of view, ignoring as it does just about everything that has been learned about heart disease and cholesterol in the past thirty years of medical science. The Lipid Research Clinics Coronary Primary Prevention Trial, for example, is considered the broadest and most expensive research project in medical history. Sponsored by the federal government, it took over ten years of systematic research and cost over $150 million. Dr. George Lundberg, editor of *The Journal of the American Medical Association* where the gargantuan study was first published, said that the study proved that even small changes in blood cholesterol levels produce dramatic changes in heart-disease rates. Dr. Charles Glueck, Director of the University of Cincinnati Lipid Research Center, one of the twelve major centers participating in the project, noted: "For every one-percent reduction in total blood cholesterol level, there is a two-percent reduction of heart-disease risk."

SOY AND BIRTH DEFECTS

One of the most alarming allegations that Fallon and Enig and other anti-soy campaigners make is that, due to the phytoestrogens in soy foods, vegetarian diets promote birth defects. They repeatedly refer to a study published in *The British*

Journal of Urology that found baby boys born to vegetarian mothers were five times more likely to suffer from hypospadias, a malformation of the penis correctable with surgery. I find this disturbing, but I know of no other study that links vegetarian diets with a higher rate of any birth defect, including hypospadias. Moreover, there are a number that show the opposite—lower rates of a variety of birth defects in babies born to vegetarian mothers. If the findings of this study are valid, however, it would be extremely important.

We certainly need more studies to determine what is going on, but after reading the actual study, I am not nearly as concerned as I was upon reading Fallon and Enig's description, because what they neglect to mention is the significant fact that the total number of baby boys in the study born with this condition to vegetarian mothers was only seven.

It's hard to know just what to make of this small and isolated study. To my eyes, it highlights how much we have yet to learn about the impact of the phytoestrogens contained in soy. Given our current state of knowledge, I think that pregnant women should largely avoid soy-based supplements. But there is no cause to conclude that vegetarian diets or soy foods are suspect in pregnancy.

Vegetarian diets have consistently shown profound benefits for pregnancy and lactation, including much lower levels of the toxic chemicals that are typically found in higher concentrations in foods higher on the food chain, most notably meat, fish, and dairy products. A report in *The New England Journal of Medicine* on the levels of contamination in human breast milk found that vegan mothers had dramatically lower levels of toxic chemicals in their milk compared with mothers in the general population. The highest level seen among these vegan mothers was actually lower than the lowest level seen in non-vegetarian mothers. In fact, the level of contamination found in the milk of the vegetarian mothers was only

1 to 2 percent as great as the level found in the milk of non-vegetarians.

Infant Soy Formula

Another of the disturbing charges made by the soy bashers is the allegation that "an infant exclusively fed soy formula receives the estrogenic equivalent (based on body weight) of at least five birth control pills per day." Soy formula, say Fallon and Enig, amounts to "birth control pills for babies."

In my view, there could be some basis here for concern. For an adult to eat soy regularly characteristically produces a reduced risk of developing breast or prostate cancer. But the same phytoestrogens that produce this effect in adults may produce very different effects in infants. "With adults, half their phytoestrogens are freed into the bloodstream to bind to estrogen receptors, which helps to fight breast cancer," explains Patricia Bertron, dietitian and Director of the Physicians Committee for Responsible Medicine. "But with infants, less than 5 percent are available to bind to receptors." There is a possibility that this could pose a risk to the sexual development of infants and children. Because the milk source makes up nearly the entire diet of infants, babies fed soy formulas may be at increased risk of harm.

These theoretical risks are quite disturbing, but they appear at this point to be merely theoretical, because we have yet to see any substantive evidence of this harm in people. There have been no reports of hormonal abnormalities in people who were fed soy formula as infants—and this includes millions of people in the past thirty years. In fact, a major study published in the August 2001 *Journal of the American Medical Association* found that infants fed soy formula grow to be just as healthy as those raised on cow's milk formulas. If the phytoestrogens in soy were affecting the reproductive system of infants fed soy formulas, then soy-fed babies would develop reproductive health problems as adults. The study evaluated 811 men and women between the ages of twenty and thirty-four who had participated in soy and cow's milk studies as infants. No significant differences were found between the groups in more than thirty health areas. The only exception was that women who had been soy-fed reported slightly longer menstrual periods (one-third of a day) than women raised on cow's milk formulas.

The debate as to which is better—formulas based on soy or cow's milk—is unresolved. Each seems to have its own dangers. What is indisputable is that babies reared on breast milk have phenomenal health advantages over babies reared on any type of formula.

Compared with babies who are fed either soy- or cow's-milk-based formulas, babies who are beast-fed for at least six months:

- Have three times fewer ear infections
- Have five times fewer urinary tract infections
- Have five times fewer serious illnesses of all kinds
- Have seven times fewer allergies
- Are fourteen times less likely to be hospitalized

The health advantages of breastfeeding are almost impossible to exaggerate. Babies who are breast-fed:

- Spit up less often
- Have less diarrhea
- Have less constipation
- Are thirty times less likely to die from Sudden Infant Death Syndrome
- Are only half as likely to develop diabetes
- Have an average I.Q. seven points higher

The health benefits of breastfeeding are life-long. As adults, people who were breast-fed:

- Have less asthma
- Have fewer allergies
- Have less diabetes
- Have fewer skin problems, including dermatitis
- Have lower risks of heart attacks and stroke
- Have lower cholesterol levels
- Have less ulcerative colitis (ulcers in the large intestines)
- Have less Crohn's disease
- Have protection from certain chronic liver diseases

The evidence that "breast is best" is utterly overwhelming. Yet the anti-soy crusader Sally Fallon evidently prefers that infants be fed cow's milk formula rather than breast milk if the mother is a vegetarian. She writes that "breast milk is best *if* the mother has consumed a . . . diet . . . rich in animal proteins and fat throughout her pregnancy and continues to do so while nursing her child."

Why would someone make a statement like that? Where are these soy antagonists coming from? What are they trying to prove?

Fallon and Enig, like Kaayla Daniel and many of the other headliners in the anti-soy campaign, are proponents of the philosophy that in order to be healthy people must eat large amounts of saturated fat from animal products. They advocate feeding puréed meat to infants. And they deplore the fact that soy products are increasingly replacing animal products in the American diet.

COW'S MILK VS. SOY MILK

Some anti-soy crusaders, most notably the U.S. dairy industry, clearly have a financial agenda. In recent years, the dairy industry has been waging war particularly against soy milk. They have attempted to keep soy beverages from being included in the milk group in the Dietary Guidelines for Americans. They have sued the manufacturers of soy beverages for using the word milk, claiming that the dairy industry alone has a right to use the term. And they have tried to keep soy beverages from being sold alongside cow's milk in the grocery aisles. A spokesperson for the National Milk Producers Federation made it clear why the industry was upset. "It is," he said, "a clear attempt to compete with dairy products."

Heaven forbid.

Meanwhile, the dairy industry has been spending hundreds of millions of dollars on ads and other forms of promotion trying to convince the public that cow's milk is vastly preferable to soy milk. For example, the Dairy Bureau claims: "Unfortified soy beverages contain only half of the phosphorus, 40 percent of the riboflavin, 10 percent of the vitamin A, (and) 3 percent of the calcium . . . found in a serving of cow's milk."

Let's look at the Dairy Bureau's claims carefully for a moment.

Only half the phosphorus: That sounds bad. But we actually get plenty of phosphorus in our diets, and possibly even too much. Providing only half the phosphorus of cow's milk is an advantage, says dietician Brenda Davis, not a disadvantage.

Only 40 percent of the riboflavin: It's true that unfortified soy milks contain only about half as much of this nutrient, also known as vitamin B2, as cow's milk. But riboflavin is plentiful in nutritional yeast and green leafy vegetables, and is found in nuts, seeds, whole grains, and legumes. So getting enough riboflavin isn't a problem for people who eat a variety of healthy foods. In fact, vegans (who consume no dairy products) consume as much, or nearly as much, of this vitamin as lacto-ovo-vegetarians and non-vegetarians. A mere teaspoon of Red Star Nutritional Yeast powder contains as much riboflavin (1.6 mg) as an entire quart of cow's milk.

Only 10 percent of the vitamin A: Vitamin A is plentiful in plant-based diets. We don't need milk to get sufficient amounts of this nutrient. In fact, vitamin A deficiency is quite rare among North Americans and Europeans who eat plant-based diets. Furthermore, vitamin A content is high in cow's milk only because it's added to it, and there is no reason it could not be added to non-dairy beverages if there were some advantage to doing so.

Only 3 percent of the calcium: Where does the dairy industry come up with this stuff? All of the most popular soy beverages sold in the United States provide vastly more calcium than the 3 percent claimed by the Dairy Bureau. Most enriched versions provide 100 percent as much. Even those soy beverages that have not been enriched provide two to nine times the calcium claimed by the Dairy Bureau.

Meanwhile, there are a few more things the dairy industry isn't telling you about the nutritional comparison between cow's milk and soy milk that you may want to keep in mind. For example:

- Cow's milk provides more than nine times as much saturated fat as soy beverages, so is far more likely to contribute to heart disease.

- Soy beverages provide more than ten times as much essential fatty acids as cow's milk, and so provide a far healthier quality of fat.

- Soy beverages are cholesterol-free, while cow's milk contains 34 mg of cholesterol per cup.

- Soy beverages lower both total and LDL ("bad") cholesterol levels, while cow's milk raises both total and LDL cholesterol levels.

- Soy beverages contain numerous protective phytochemicals that may protect against chronic illnesses like heart disease and osteoporosis. Cow's milk contains no phytochemicals.

FRANKENSOY

Still, there are legitimate questions about soy. To my mind, by far the most disturbing one stems from the fact that 90 percent of the U.S. soybean crop today is genetically engineered. These are beans that have been genetically altered to enable the growing plants to withstand being sprayed with Monsanto's Roundup weed killer. Because so much Roundup is used on these crops, the residue levels in the harvested crops greatly exceed what, until very recently, was the allowable legal limit. For the technology to be commercially viable, the FDA had to triple the allowable residue of Roundup's active ingredients that can remain on the crop. Many scientists have protested that permitting increased residues to enable a company's success reflects an attitude in which corporate interests are given higher priority than public safety, but the increased levels have remained in force.

While Roundup has been shown to cause reproductive disorders and birth defects in a large number of animal studies, its impact on humans is far less understood. But a laboratory study done in France in 2005 found that Roundup caused the death of human placental cells. And a 2009 study found that Roundup caused total cell death in human umbilical, embryonic, and placental cells within twenty-four hours.

It's hard to avoid the suspicion that eating genetically engineered soybeans could pose serious health risks to people. In 2001, *The Los Angeles Times* published an exposé revealing that, prior to being granted FDA approval, Monsanto's own research had raised many questions about the safety of their Roundup Ready soybeans. Remarkably, the FDA did not call for more testing before allowing these soybeans to flood the marketplace. Since 90 percent of the soybeans grown in the United States are now Monsanto's Roundup Ready variety, and because soy is contained in such a wide array of processed foods, tens of millions of people are unknowingly eating these inadequately researched foods daily. It's a mass experiment, except that there is no control group. Data is not being systematically collected and virtually the entire human population is the guinea pig.

According to Monsanto's own tests, Roundup Ready soybeans contain 29 percent less of the brain nutrient choline and 27 percent more trypsin inhibitor (the potential allergen that interferes with protein digestion) than normal soybeans. Soy products are often prescribed and consumed for their phytoestrogen content, but, according to the company's tests, the genetically altered soybeans have lower levels of phenylalanine, an essential amino acid that affects levels of phytoestrogens. And levels of lectins, which are most likely the culprit in soy allergies, are nearly double in the transgenic variety.

Compared with regular soybeans, the genetically engineered beans have more of the very things that are problematic, and less of the very things that are beneficial. Furthermore, there is growing evidence that Roundup Ready soybeans disrupt the bacterial milieu of the human gastrointestinal tract.

In 2011, one of the nation's senior scientists, Dr. Don Huber, Professor Emeritus at Purdue University, informed Secretary of Agriculture Tom Vilsack of a dire new development. A new pathogen had been discovered that may already be doing irreparable harm to both plants and animals. Dr. Huber pleaded with Vilsack to understand:

> It is widespread, very serious, and is in much higher concentrations in Roundup Ready soybeans and corn. . . . This could result in a collapse of U.S. soy and corn export markets and significant disruption of domestic food and feed supplies. . . . For the past 40 years, I have been a scientist in the professional and military agencies that evaluate and prepare for natural and manmade biological threats, including germ warfare and disease outbreaks. Based on this experience, I believe the threat we are facing from this pathogen is unique and of a high risk status. In layman's terms, it . . . is an emergency.

Recognizing that virtually all U.S. beef cattle, dairy cows, and pigs are fed Roundup Ready soy, Huber went on to write:

> The pathogen may explain the escalating frequency of infertility and spontaneous abortions over the past few years in U.S. cattle, dairy, swine, and horse operations. These include recent reports of infertility rates in dairy heifers of over 20 percent, and spontaneous abortions in cattle as high as 45 percent. . . .

> It is well-documented that [Roundup's primary active ingredient] glyphosate promotes soil pathogens and is already implicated with the increase of more than 40 plant diseases; it dismantles plant defenses by chelating vital nutrients; and it reduces the bioavailability of nutrients in feed, which in turn can cause animal disorders. . . .

I have studied plant pathogens for more than 50 years. We are now seeing an unprecedented trend of increasing plant and animal diseases and disorders. This pathogen may be instrumental to understanding and solving this problem. It deserves immediate attention with significant resources to avoid a general collapse of our critical agricultural infrastructure.

There is a very real danger hidden today in the world of soy, but it is not what the anti-soy brigade would have us believe. While they have been saying that soy foods are hazardous to human health, they have been missing the real danger. Monsanto's Roundup Ready soybeans now represent almost the entire U.S. soy crop.

Here is one of the strongest arguments ever made for organic foods: The only way to ensure that the soy foods you eat are not Roundup Ready is to be sure that they are organically grown.

TO SOY OR NOT TO SOY

While soy foods have much to offer, they have certainly been heavily over-promoted at times. As a result, some people have gathered the impression that as long as they eat enough soy, they don't have to worry about the rest of their diet and lifestyle. This is a dangerous and mistaken belief. Just as taking vitamins can't atone for a poor diet, consuming soy can't make up for a diet that's otherwise poor. Nor can it compensate for a lack of exercise or other destructive lifestyle habits.

The hype has also made us forget something important. We are eating soy products today at levels never before seen in history. Advances in food technology have made it possible to isolate soy proteins, isoflavones, and other substances found in the bean, and add them to all kinds of foods where they've never been before. The number of processed and manufactured foods that contain soy ingredients today is astounding. It can be hard to find foods that don't contain soy flour, soy oil, lecithin (extracted from soy oil and used as an emulsifier in high-fat products), soy-protein isolates and concentrates, textured vegetable protein (TVP), hydrolyzed vegetable protein (usually made from soy), or unidentified vegetable oils. Most of what is labeled "vegetable oil" in the U.S. is actually soy oil. And most of our soy products are now genetically engineered.

This has never before been done in human history. It is an experiment that should be undertaken, if at all, with great humility, watchfulness, and caution. Instead, under the influence of an almost mystical belief in soy's virtues, we've tended to fall prey to an illusion that has haunted American culture in all kinds of ways—the illusion that if a little is good, then surely more must be better.

The anti-soy crusaders, on the other hand, tell us that any amount of soy is too much. They are correct that there are substances in soy that, if eaten in too high a concentration, can cause problems. The reality, however, is that this is true of almost all foods. In fact, if you made it your policy to eat no food that contained substances that can, in large enough concentrations, cause damage, there would be literally nothing left for you to eat.

It's true that soybeans contain substances that, in excess, can be harmful. But to imply, as some do, that eating soy foods poses a risk to human health is twisting and distorting the evidence. There are dangers in eating a diet based entirely on soybeans. But, then, the same can be said for broccoli or any other healthy food. This is one of the reasons why varied diets are so important. Diversity protects. For most people under most circumstances, soy products are a healthful addition to a balanced diet that includes plenty of vegetables, whole grains, seeds, nuts, fruits, and other legumes. For most people, substituting soy foods for some of the animal foods they now eat is one of the healthiest dietary changes they can make.

In my view, the best way to take advantage of soy's health benefits is to follow the example of traditional Asian diets. In general, Asians eating their traditional diets have tended to be healthier and live longer than Americans. The Okinawa Japanese, the longest-living people in the world, average one to two servings of soy each day. They have traditionally eaten regular but moderate amounts of whole soy foods like tofu, soy milk, and edamame, as well as the fermented versions, tamari and miso. These are the soy foods that I prefer to eat—rather than the soy products made with soy-protein isolates and concentrates, hydrolyzed soy protein, partially hydrogenated soy oil, etc. Whole soy foods are more natural, and are the soy foods that have nourished entire civilizations for centuries.

For me, the best of the bean includes foods like:

Tofu: The soaking process traditionally used to make tofu reduces the trypsin inhibitors and phytates. High in protein, tofu has a bland and neutral taste, and can be added to all kinds of foods. As with all soy products, get organic if you can.

Tempeh: Extremely high in protein and fiber, and produced in a way that greatly lowers trypsin inhibitors and phytates, tempeh is, from a nutritional perspective, an ideal way to eat soybeans. Most people feel it needs considerable seasoning to taste good.

Miso: Widely used as a salty condiment and a basis for soups, miso is a potent probiotic, containing many kinds of friendly bacteria that are beneficial to the intestinal tract. The fermentation process used to make miso deactivates the trypsin inhibitors and phytates.

Tamari (Shoyu): This is a fermented soy sauce that is very flavorful and salty.

Soy milk: Often called soy "beverages," or soy "drinks," because the dairy industry refuses to allow them to use the word "milk." Trypsin inhibitors and phytates are low. I prefer the brands made with whole soybeans, and avoid those made with soy protein or soy-milk powder. (There are also milks made from rice, almonds, and oats that offer their own advantages over cow's milk.)

Soy nuts and soy-nut butter: These are particular favorites with many children. Roasting helps reduce phytate levels.

Edamame: This is a green vegetable soybean harvested while immature, so that the seeds fill 80 to 90 percent of the pod. Cooked for about fifteen minutes in lightly salted boiling water, it's served as a snack, mixed with vegetables, or added to salads or soups.

Soy ice cream (non-dairy frozen dessert): These may not technically belong on a list of the healthiest of ways to eat soy, but I must admit I've got a weakness for them. I eat the ones made with organic beans and/or organic soy milk, and not those (like Tofutti) made with soy proteins or soy-protein isolates. (There are also frozen desserts made from coconut milk and other plant foods that offer advantages over cow's-milk ice cream.)

THE MIDDLE ROAD

Genetically engineered soybeans present us with a historically unprecedented problem, and argue strongly for organics. Even if you eat only organically grown soy, becoming a soy-a-holic and automatically downing anything made from soybeans is not the road to health. But neither is shunning and stigmatizing soy foods.

The anti-soy crusade has needlessly frightened many away from a food source that has long been a boon to humankind— a food source that can, if we are respectful of our bodies and of nature, nourish and bless us in countless ways.

5

Does Soy Cause Alzheimer's?

THERE IS ONE MORE ACCUSATION against soy that deserves attention. You may have seen headlines proclaiming that "tofu shrinks brains," or heard that soy consumption causes Alzheimer's disease. These sensational allegations began appearing after a study was published in April 2000 in *The Journal of the American College of Nutrition.*

The study, conducted in Hawaii by Dr. Lon White and his associates, was part of the Honolulu Heart Study. Looking at the diets and the risk of dementia in Japanese men residing in Hawaii, the study found that men who ate the most tofu during their mid-forties to mid-sixties were more likely to develop dementia and Alzheimer's as they grew older.

The correlation between tofu and cognitive decline was strong, and could not be explained by confounding factors like age, education, and obesity. In this study, men who had eaten two or more servings of tofu per week in midlife were 2.4 times more likely than men who rarely or never ate tofu to become senile or forgetful by old age. Even the wives of men who ate tofu showed more signs of dementia.

This was startling and completely unexpected. Soy has been shown repeatedly to lower cholesterol levels, and high cholesterol levels have long been intimately linked to increased risk for Alzheimer's.

And for soy eaters, it was frightening. If that's all you know, it looks pretty bad for soy.

But that's not all we know. We also know, for example, that dementia rates are lower in Asian countries, where soy intake is high, than in Western countries. We know that the Japanese lifestyle, with its high soy intake, has long been associated with longer life span and better cognition in old age. And we know that Seventh Day Adventists, many of whom consume soy foods their whole lives, have less dementia in old age than the general population.

If tofu consumption increases Alzheimer's incidence, then there would be more Alzheimer's in Japan than in Hawaii, because more tofu is eaten in Japan. But, in fact, the reverse is true.

What, then, could have been the cause of these mysterious findings?

People with Alzheimer's disease characteristically have higher levels of aluminum in their brains. Many studies have shown a link between increased levels of aluminum consumption and the risk of Alzheimer's disease. Higher levels of aluminum in drinking water, for example, typically produce higher rates of the disease. When a physician practicing in Hawaii, Bill Harris, subsequently had soy products made in Hawaii and those from the mainland tested and compared for their aluminum levels, the levels of aluminum in the Hawaii products were found to be significantly higher. Could it be that the aluminum used in the refining of some soy products in Hawaii is the actual culprit? To my knowledge, no other study has found a link between soy consumption and Alzheimer's, but many studies have supported the link between aluminum and the disease.

Moreover, the Honolulu Heart Study has some very real limitations. There are many lifestyle factors for which it did not control. The researchers who conducted the study were the first to acknowledge that tofu consumption may be a marker for some other factor that negatively affects cognitive function. This would make tofu an innocent bystander. Results of many other studies suggest that this is the case.

A number of clinical studies have shown that soy (and isoflavones from soy) is actually beneficial for cognition. In one study, published in the journal *Psychopharmacology* in 2001, young adult men and women who ate a high-soy diet experienced substantial improvements in short-term and long-term memory and in mental flexibility. Other studies have found that isoflavone supplements from soy improve cognitive function in postmenopausal women.

While the Honolulu Heart Study is concerning, it appears to be an aberration. More than ten years have passed since the Honolulu Heart Study was published, and there have been no further long-term studies showing any relationship between soy and dementia in humans. There have, however, been a number of clinical trials that have found soy to improve memory and other forms of cognitive function.

Meanwhile, an ever-growing number of studies are pointing to the practical and proven steps you can take to lower your risk of Alzheimer's and help assure that you will retain the ability to think clearly throughout the length of your days.

What are these steps? Let's find out.

EXERCISE: EVEN MORE IMPORTANT THAN YOU MAY THINK

You may be surprised to learn that many studies have found that regular physical exercise plays an essential role in preventing Alzheimer's disease. For example, a five-year study published in *Archives of Neurology* in March 2001 found that people with the highest activity levels were only half as likely as inactive people to develop Alzheimer's disease, and were also substantially less likely to suffer any other form of dementia or mental impairment. Even those who engaged in light or moderate exercise had significant reductions in their risk for Alzheimer's and other forms of mental decline. The study concluded that the more people exercise, the healthier their brains remain as they grow older.

Three years later, in September 2004, *The Journal of the American Medical Association* published a series of studies further confirming that regular exercise helps preserve clear thinking even at advanced ages. One study found that women aged seventy and older who had higher levels of physical activity scored better on cognitive performance tests and showed less cognitive decline than women who were less active. Even walking for only two hours a week at an easy pace made a marked difference, although the most marked benefit was found in women who walked six hours a week. Another study found that older men who walked two miles a day had only half the rate of dementia found among men who walked less than a quarter-mile a day.

Two years later, a study published in *The Annals of Internal Medicine* found that older adults who exercise three or more times a week have a 30 to 40 percent lower risk of developing dementia than their more sedentary counterparts.

UNEXPECTED BENEFITS OF A PLANT-STRONG DIET

Meanwhile, a plethora of studies are telling us that there is something even more important than exercise in preventing Alzheimer's disease. And that—drum roll please—is a healthy plant-strong diet.

Why? There are many reasons. One is that plant-strong diets are high in antioxidants. Antioxidants are substances that keep you young and healthy by increasing immune function, decreasing the risk of infection and cancer, and, most important, protecting against free-radical damage. Free radicals are cellular desperadoes that play a pivotal role in the aging process. Their damage takes a toll on virtually every organ and system in the aging human body. This, in turn, sets the stage for all sorts of degenerative diseases, including Alzheimer's. Antioxidants help to prevent this damage by neutralizing free radicals.

Antioxidants are found in fresh vegetables, whole grains, fresh fruits, and legumes like soy. If your diet is high in antioxidants, your risk of many age-associated diseases—including dementia, cancer, heart disease, macular degeneration, and cataracts—decreases.

Another reason plant-strong diets help prevent Alzheimer's is that they help you to stay slim. How important is that? In 2004, Dr. Miia Kivipelto of the Karolinska Institute in Sweden told an international conference on Alzheimer's disease in Philadelphia of his twenty-one-year study, which found that people who were obese in middle age were twice as likely to develop dementia when they got old as those who were of normal weight. For those who also had high cholesterol and high blood pressure in middle age, the risk of dementia was six times higher.

Plant-strong diets also help you stay mentally clear as you grow older by keeping your homocysteine levels low. Homocysteine is a toxic amino acid, a breakdown product of protein metabolism that has been strongly linked to Alzheimer's and also to heart attacks, strokes, depression, and a type of blindness. Even small elevations in homocysteine can significantly increase the risk for these conditions.

Blood levels of homocysteine are typically higher in people whose diets are high in meat and low in leafy vegetables, whole grains, legumes, and fruits. Plant-strong diets provide folic acid and other B vitamins that help the body get rid of homocysteine.

One study found that the incidence of Alzheimer's was a staggering 3.3 times greater among people whose blood folic acid levels were in the lowest one-third range, and 4.3 times greater for those with the lowest levels of vitamin B12.

In 2001, the journal *Neurology* published the results of a three-year Swedish study of 370 healthy elderly adults. The study found that those with even slightly lower levels of vitamin B12 and folic acid had twice the risk of developing Alzheimer's disease compared with those with normal levels.

Folic acid and the B vitamins, remember, are crucial because they help to maintain low homocysteine levels. On October 18, 1998, Dr. David Smith and his colleagues from Oxford University presented their findings to the American Medical Association's annual Science Reporters' Conference. Their study, published in *Archives of Neurology* the following month, found that the risk of getting Alzheimer's disease was 4.5 times greater when blood homocysteine levels were in the highest one-third.

A study of 3,000 Chicago residents aged sixty-five and older published in *The Journal of Neurology, Neurosurgery and Psychiatry* in 2004 found that those with the lowest intake of dietary niacin (vitamin B3) were 70 percent more likely to develop Alzheimer's than those with a higher intake, and their rate of cognitive decline was twice as fast. The take-home message is simple: Eat greens. The best dietary sources of niacin are dark-green leafy vegetables.

Vegans in particular need to understand that adequate levels of vitamin B12 are necessary for folic acid to carry out its functions effectively. The most common sources of B12 for vegans include supplements (a pleasant-tasting supplement typically costs a few pennies per week), and fortified products including soy milk and nutritional yeast.

But it is meat-eaters who are most at risk for high homocysteine levels, because animal foods (and meat in particular) tend to contribute to the production of homocysteine. *One study found that subjects who ate meat as their main source of protein were nearly three times as likely to develop dementia as their vegetarian counterparts.* A survey of the medical literature on diet and Alzheimer's noted how frequently a meat-centered diet raises homocysteine levels. The report was aptly entitled "Losing Your Mind for the Sake of a Burger."

In our society, we often take for granted that aging will bring restricted short-term memory and diminished mental faculties. A visit to most nursing homes demonstrates how commonly and how markedly people in our society experience cognitive decline as they age.

But there is good science to show that we can experience clear thinking well into our later years. It turns out that it is not soy consumption, but the standard American high-saturated-fat diet—low in vegetables and fruits and whole grains, and thus low in brain-preserving antioxidants—that is primarily responsible for the unhealthy outcomes we so often see in our elderly.

If you eat consciously, exercise regularly, and seek to enjoy every precious moment of your life, you won't be another one of the people who end up lamenting: "If I had known I was going to live this long, I would have taken better care of myself."

6

It's Not about Size, It's about Health: Obesity and Food Choices

WE CAN, AS A SOCIETY, be astoundingly cruel to people who are obese. They may be creative, caring, and hopeful people, but we don't see that. Far too often, we see only their weight.

What does it say about us that we act as though you can take the measure of a person by the size bathing suit he or she wears?

Maybe this partially explains why obese people are flocking to a restaurant outside Phoenix, Arizona whose name—and I am not making this up—is the Heart Attack Grill. The restaurant, which seats 100, is often packed. It offers what owner Jon Basso calls "an environment of acceptance to overweight customers who are typically demonized by society."

At this restaurant, however, it's a little more than acceptance. The Heart Attack Grill literally celebrates obesity. Customers who are over 350 pounds eat for free. A scale is strategically placed at the center of the restaurant so that other diners can watch the weigh-ins. When customers exceed 350 pounds, says the restaurant's owner, "Everybody applauds and cheers for them. A big smile comes over their faces, and for once they are finally accepted. They are not picked on here."

It's all made to seem sexy, too. Waitresses, all of them young and slender, are dressed as scantily clad nurses, wearing high heels, thigh-high stockings, and skimpy outfits revealing lots of cleavage.

It sounds like fun.

Except when it isn't.

In 2011, the 575-pound spokesman for the Heart Attack Grill, a 29-year-old man named Blair River, died—not from a heart attack, but from pneumonia. He had been the public face of the restaurant and the star of its advertising. He was also the single father of a five-year-old girl.

At nearly 600 pounds, Blair River ate all his meals free at the restaurant.

Heart Attack Grill owner Jon Basso did not deny the link between the young man's excessive weight and his tragically premature death. "I hired him to promote my food," said Basso, "[but his] life was cut short because he carried extra weight." Ironically, the restaurant's motto is "Food Worth Dying For."

Of course, no one is forcing anyone to eat at the Heart Attack Grill or to stuff themselves full of unhealthy food. It's a free country—in theory anyway—and we're free to eat ourselves to death if we want to do so.

Some would say that the Heart Attack Grill steps over a line, to the point of enabling dangerous food addictions. There is certainly nothing remotely resembling healthy on the menu. Customers can purchase cigarettes, but only the non-filtered type. On the wall are prominent displays advertising menu items like "Quadruple Bypass Burgers" that carry 8,000 calories, and "Flatliner Fries" that are deep-fried in pure lard. Perhaps joking, owner Basso says, "We're in the front lines of the battle against anorexia."

But Blair River's death is no joke. And it would be a mistake to make light of the medical consequences of obesity. The CDC tells us that obese people have a substantially higher risk for not only heart attacks, but also for diabetes, most cancers, and many other types of cardiovascular disease.

Heart Attack Grill owner Basso doesn't plan any changes on account of Blair's death. Scantily-clad waitresses will still regularly exhort customers to eat all they can. He's making money and thinks the restaurant is great fun.

But is it funny that we have become the most obese society in the history of the world? Two-thirds of the residents of the United States are now either overweight or obese. So many children are developing the most common type of diabetes that medical authorities have had to change the name of the disease. What was formerly called "adult-onset diabetes" is now called "type-2 diabetes" and now accounts for 90 percent of the diabetes in the country. Its incidence in children is skyrocketing.

It's easy to point our fingers and pass judgment. We can blame fast-food companies that aggressively market unhealthy foods to children, we can blame people who overeat because of a lack of will power, and we can blame parents for feeding their children poorly. We can blame harmful ingredients like trans-fats and high-fructose corn syrup, and we can blame the pressures of modern life that turn people into addicts of one kind or another.

We can play the blame game *ad infinitum*, but whom does that help? Does it help those with weight problems that leave them vulnerable to disease and prone to feelings of shame?

What if we were instead to learn from people who have taken the arduous, difficult, and ultimately joyful journey from obesity to health?

Recently, I have had the wonderful good fortune to become friends with a young woman named Natala Constantine and her husband Matt. They've been married for seven and a half years. At their wedding, Natala was morbidly obese.

She knew something about the abuse endured by obese people in our society. By then, she had lost track of the number of times she had been humiliated in public, called ugly names by strangers, and physically hurt by people who felt entitled to treat her as less than human because of her weight.

People constantly told Natala she was lucky Matt had fallen in love with her, and that he must be amazing to be able to look past her weight.

A week after the wedding, she was diagnosed with severe diabetes. Her blood had become so acidic that her organs were shutting down, and doctors seriously doubted she would survive. She was twenty-five years old.

Five years later, Natala was taking up to thirteen different medications and as much as 200 units of insulin a day. She ate what many people would call a healthy diet—lots of animal protein and almost no carbohydrates. She had been told that a diet high in animal protein was the only way she could control her diabetes, but it wasn't working. She was working out at a gym for two to three hours a day, but at 5´2˝ tall, she weighed close to 400 pounds.

When Natala developed an infection in her right calf, doctors told her that part of her lower right leg might need to be amputated. But then a friend, whom Natala described to me as "a vegan and into yoga," suggested that she consider a natural approach to her diabetes, and that she should start to think of food as medicine. "I wanted to smash her," Natala admits. "How dare she suggest something so simple! Didn't she know that I had been to the best doctors? That I was on the best diet? That I was working out?"

But Natala did take her friend's advice to heart, and decided to go on what she calls a "100 percent healthy plant-strong diet."

"For the first three weeks," she says, "I felt as though I was ridding myself of much more than animal products. Food had a hold on me that I could not even conceptualize prior to those three weeks. I would sit in my car and cry outside of sub shops, just wanting a tuna melt."

It was very rough, but Natala stayed with it and the results were nothing short of miraculous. In thirty days, she was off all insulin.

The physicians she was seeing for her diabetes took a look at her numbers, were amazed, and wanted to know how she had done it. "I told them I had adopted a completely plant-based diet. They didn't seem surprised at all, and told me that plant-based diets were helping to reverse diabetes. When I asked why they had not suggested it, they told me because it isn't practical."

Aghast, she asked her doctor, "Do you think it's practical to be thirty years old and lose a leg?"

She walked out of that doctor's office and never went back. "Everything changed from that moment," she recalls. "I slowly decreased all the other diabetes medicines I was on. I lowered my blood cholesterol without drugs. I lowered my blood pressure without drugs. I corrected my hormonal problems without drugs. Many diabetics go blind, but I reversed the nerve damage in my eyes. And that infection in my leg? It completely healed. The arthritis in my feet? It went away."

Today, Natala Constantine has lost almost 200 pounds, is medicine-free, and continues to make great strides toward her ideal weight. Her diabetes is in complete remission. I've met her and I can attest that she is one of the happiest and most radiant people you could hope to meet. A concert violinist, she exudes joy.

And her husband, Matt? While Natala was dealing with diabetes, he was not only obese, but also suffered from severe food allergies. Eating a few tomatoes sent him to the emergency room. His food allergies dominated his life. And now?

His improvement, on a 100 percent healthy plant-strong diet, is almost as miraculous as his wife's. A concert pianist, he has lost ninety pounds and is now at a healthy weight; his food allergies are entirely behind him.

It's quite a world we live in it, isn't it? On the one hand, we have the Heart Attack Grill, whose 575-pound spokesman died at the age of twenty-nine. On the other, we have people like Natala and Matt Constantine, who have taken a different path.

We live in a society that tends to stigmatize the obese cruelly. The Heart Attack Grill represents one form of response. It can feel temporarily empowering to turn shame into defiance. When society points its finger at you, blaming you and denying its own illness, there is a natural urge to send a message back to society with your middle finger.

But is there a healthier alternative? What about entering what Veronica Monet calls "the shame-free zone" while making a commitment to greater well-being and happiness? What about refusing to internalize society's negative messages, and instead building a healthy life of joy, confidence, and beauty?

Cutting back on heavily sweetened beverages like sodas and juice-like drinks is a good place to start. Eating fewer processed foods and more whole foods is another good step. Getting exercise helps a lot. And the more of your nutrients you can get from plant sources, the better.

Eat a healthy plant-strong diet, and your body will thank you for the rest of your life.

After the article on which this chapter is based was published on *Huffington Post*, I received many emails from people who told me of their weight-loss experiences. Here are just two that brought me joy to read. Gary Paulson wrote:

> Just read your article in the *Huffington Post*, and I wanted to take a moment and tell you that it was both informative

and enjoyable. I recently went through my own battle with weight loss and was able to lose almost 200 pounds with the assistance of a low-calorie, high-protein plant-based diet. One of the things I truly enjoyed about your article is your attempt to get past the infinite blame game, and open up to an honest dialogue about some potential solutions for the obesity crisis currently facing America. Moreover, you did so in a way that was both humane and sensitive to those currently struggling with weight issues, and all the stigmas that go along with it.

Actress-singer Kate Chapman used to get only the "fat lady" parts. Now that she's lost weight and is half her former size, she has the stamina to perform show after show and dance from curtain to curtain; she is taking Broadway by storm. She wrote:

> Thank you so much for your article in *Huffington Post* today. I, too, have reversed obesity by eating a mostly plant diet, and for the first time in forty years, I don't struggle with my weight. Three years ago, I finished my 100 pound weight loss, and have maintained the entire loss since then, without effort. I thank you for writing what you did. I was in Phoenix for work last year and saw the Heart Attack Grill. It made me sad then, and makes me sadder now. Thank you for helping to get the word out that those of us who have reversed the trend for ourselves really can help others to lead healthier, happier, and less encumbered lives. Maybe if we all work together, we can turn it around.

7

The Skinny on Grass-fed Beef

A LOT OF PEOPLE TODAY, horrified by how animals are treated in factory farms and feedlots, and wanting to lower their ecological footprint, are looking for healthier alternatives. As a result, there is a decided trend toward pasture-raised animals. One former vegetarian, *San Francisco Chronicle* columnist Mark Morford, says he now eats meat, but only "grass-fed and organic and sustainable as possible, reverentially and deeply gratefully, and in small amounts."

Sales of grass-fed and organic beef are rising rapidly. Ten years ago, there were only about fifty grass-fed cattle operations left in the U.S. Now there are thousands.

How much difference does it make? Is grass-fed really better? If so, in what ways, and how much?

If you read on, you'll see why I've concluded that grass-fed is indeed better. But then, almost anything would be. Putting beef cattle in feedlots and feeding them grain may actually be one of the dumbest ideas in the history of Western civilization.

Cattle (like sheep, deer, and other grazing animals) are endowed with the ability to convert grasses that we humans cannot digest into flesh that we can digest. They can do this because, unlike humans who possess only one stomach, they are ruminants. They possess a second stomach called a rumen—a roughly forty-five-gallon fermentation tank in which resident bacteria convert cellulose into protein and fats.

In today's feedlots, however, cows fed corn and other grains are eating food that human can eat, and they are quite inefficiently converting it into meat. Since it takes anywhere from seven to sixteen pounds of grain to make a pound of feedlot beef, we actually get far less food out than we put in. It's a protein factory in reverse.

And we do this on a massive scale, while nearly a billion people on our planet do not have enough to eat.

FEEDLOT REALITY

How has a system that is so wasteful come to be? Feedlots and other CAFOs (Confined Animal Feeding Operations) are not the inevitable product of agricultural progress, nor are they the result of market forces. They are instead the result of public policies that massively favor large-scale feed-lots to the detriment of family farms.

From 1997 to 2005, for example, taxpayer-subsidized grain prices saved feedlots and other CAFOs about $35 billion. This subsidy is so large that it reduced the price CAFOs pay for animal feed to a tiny fraction of what it would otherwise have been. Cattle operations that raise animals exclusively on pasture land, however, derive no benefit from the subsidy.

Federal policies also give CAFOs billions of dollars to address their pollution problems, which arise because they confine so many animals, often tens of thousands, in a small area. Small farmers raising cattle on pasture do not have this problem in the first place. If feedlots and other CAFOs were required to pay the price of handling their animal waste in an environmentally healthy manner—if they were made to pay to prevent or to clean up the pollution they create—they wouldn't be dominating the U.S. meat industry the way they are today. But instead, we have had farm policies that require the taxpayers to foot the bill. Such policies have made feedlots and other CAFOs feasible, but only by fleecing the public.

Traditionally, all beef was grass-fed beef, but we've turned that completely upside down. Now, thanks to our misguided policies, our beef supply is almost all feedlot beef.

Thanks to government subsidies, it's cheaper, and it's also faster. Seventy-five years ago, steers were slaughtered at the age of four or five years old. Today's steers, however, grow so fast on the grain they are fed that they can be butchered much younger, typically when they are only 14 to 16 months old.

All beef cattle spend the first few months of their lives on pasture or rangeland, where they graze on forage crops like grass or alfalfa. But then nearly all are fattened—or as the industry likes to call it "finished"—in feedlots where they eat grain. You can't take a beef calf from a birth weight of 80 pounds to 1,200 pounds in a little more than a year on grass. That kind of unnaturally fast weight gain takes enormous quantities of corn, soy-based protein supplements, antibiotics, and other drugs, including growth hormones.

Under current farm policies, switching a cow from grass to corn makes economic sense, but it is still profoundly disturbing to the animal's digestive system. It can actually kill a steer if not done gradually and if the animal is not continually fed antibiotics.

Author (and small-scale cattleman) Michael Pollan describes what happens to cows when they are taken off of pastures and put into feedlots and fed corn:

> Perhaps the most serious thing that can go wrong with a ruminant on corn is feedlot bloat. The rumen is always producing copious amounts of gas, which is normally expelled by belching during rumination. But when the

diet contains too much starch and too little roughage, rumination all but stops, and a layer of foamy slime that can trap gas forms in the rumen. The rumen inflates like a balloon, pressing against the animal's lungs. Unless action is promptly taken to relieve the pressure (usually by forcing a hose down the animal's esophagus), the cow suffocates.

A corn diet can also give a cow acidosis. Unlike our own highly acidic stomachs, the normal pH of a rumen is neutral. Corn makes it unnaturally acidic, however, causing a kind of bovine heartburn, which in some cases can kill the animal but usually just makes it sick. Acidotic animals go off their feed, pant and salivate excessively, paw at their bellies and eat dirt. The condition can lead to diarrhea, ulcers, bloat, liver disease, and a general weakening of the immune system that leaves the animal vulnerable to everything from pneumonia to feedlot polio.

Putting beef cattle in feedlots and giving them corn is not only unnatural and dangerous for the cows. It also has profound medical consequences for us, and this is true whether or not we eat their flesh. Feedlot beef as we know it today would be impossible if it weren't for the routine and continual feeding of antibiotics to these animals. This leads directly and inexorably to the development of antibiotic-resistant bacteria. These new "superbugs" are increasingly rendering our antibiotics ineffective for treating disease in humans.

Further, it is the commercial meat industry's practice of keeping cattle in feedlots and feeding them grain that is responsible for the heightened prevalence of deadly E. coli 0157:H7 bacteria. When cattle are grain-fed, their intestinal tracts become far more acidic, which favors the growth of pathogenic E. coli bacteria that can kill people who eat undercooked hamburger.

It's not widely known, but E. coli 0157:H7 has only recently appeared on the scene. It was first identified in the 1980s, but now this pathogen can be found in the intestines of almost all feedlot cattle in the U.S. Even less widely recognized is that the practice of feeding corn and other grains to cattle has created the perfect conditions for forms of E. Coli and other microbes—microbes that can, and do, kill us—to come into being.

Prior to the advent of feedlots, the microbes that resided in the intestines of cows were adapted to a neutral pH environment. As a result, if they got into meat, it didn't usually cause much of a problem because the microbes perished in the acidic environment of the human stomach. But the digestive tract of the modern feedlot animal has changed. It is now nearly as acidic as our own. In this new, man-made environment, strains of E. coli and other pathogens have developed that can survive our stomach acids, and go on to kill us. As Michael Pollan puts it: "By acidifying a cow's gut with corn, we have broken down one of our food chain's barriers to infections."

CORN-FED VS. GRASS-FED: NUTRITION, TASTE, AND THE ENVIRONMENT

Many of us think of "corn-fed" beef as nutritionally superior, but it isn't. A corn-fed cow does develop well-marbled flesh, but this is simply saturated fat that can't be trimmed off. Grass-fed meat, on the other hand, is lower both in overall fat and in artery-clogging saturated fat. A sirloin steak from a grain-fed feedlot steer has more than double the total fat of a similar cut from a grass-fed steer. In its less-than-infinite wisdom, however, the USDA continues to grade beef in a way that rewards marbling with intra-muscular fat.

Grass-fed beef is not only lower in overall fat and in saturated fat; it has the added advantage of providing more omega-3 fats. These crucial healthy fats are most plentiful in flaxseeds and fish, and are also found in walnuts and soybeans, and in meat from animals that have grazed on omega-3-rich grass. When cattle are taken off grass, however, and shipped to a feedlot to be fattened on grain, they immediately begin losing the omega-3s they have stored in their tissues. A grass-fed steak typically has about twice as many omega-3s as a grain-fed steak.

In addition to being higher in healthy omega-3s, meat from pastured cattle is also up to four times higher in vitamin E than meat from feedlot cattle, and much higher in conjugated linoleic acid (CLA), a nutrient associated with lower cancer risk.

The higher omega-3 levels and other differences in fatty-acid composition are certainly a nutritional advantage for grass-fed beef, but this comes with a culinary cost. These differences contribute to flavors and odors in grass-fed meat that some people find undesirable. Taste-panel participants have found the meat from grass-fed animals to be characterized by "off-flavors including ammonia, gamey, bitter, liverish, old, rotten, and sour."

Even the people who market grass-fed beef say this is true. Joshua Appleton, the owner of Fleisher's Grass-fed and Organic Meats in Kingston, New York says: "Grass-fed beef has a hard flavor profile for a country that's been raised on corn-fed beef."

Unlike cows in a feedlot, animals on a pasture move around. This exercise creates muscle tone, and the resulting beef can taste a little chewier than many people prefer. Grass-fed beef doesn't provide the "melt-in-your-mouth" sensation that the modern meat-eater has come to prefer.

In addition to its nutritional advantages, there are also environmental benefits to grass-fed beef. According to David Pimentel, a Cornell ecologist who specializes in agriculture and energy, the corn we feed our feedlot cattle accounts for a staggering amount of fossil-fuel energy. Growing the corn used to feed livestock takes vast quantities of chemical fertilizer, which in turn takes vast quantities of oil. Because of this dependence on petroleum, Pimentel says, a typical steer will in effect consume 284 gallons of oil in its lifetime. Comments Michael Pollan:

> We have succeeded in industrializing the beef calf, transforming what was once a solar-powered ruminant into the very last thing we need: another fossil-fuel machine.

In addition to consuming less energy, grass-fed beef has another environmental advantage—it is far less polluting. In pastures, the animals' wastes drop onto the land, becoming nutrients for the next cycle of crops. In feedlots and other forms of factory farming, however, the animals' wastes build up in enormous quantities, becoming a staggering source of water and air pollution.

From a humanitarian perspective, there is yet another advantage to pastured animal products. The animals themselves are not forced to live in confinement. The cruelties of modern factory farming are so severe that you don't have to be a vegetarian or an animal rights activist to find the conditions intolerable and a violation of the human-animal bond. Pastured livestock are not forced to endure the miseries of factory farming. They are not cooped up in cages barely larger than their own bodies, or packed together like sardines for months on end standing knee-deep in their own manure.

GRASS-FED IS NOT ORGANIC

It's important to remember that organic is not the same as grass-fed. Natural food stores often sell organic beef and dairy products that are hormone- and antibiotic-free. These products come from animals that were fed organically grown grain, but that typically still spent most of their lives—or, in the case of dairy cows, perhaps their whole lives—in feedlots. The sad reality is that almost all the organic beef and organic dairy products sold in the U.S. today come from feedlots.

Just as organic does not mean grass-fed, grass-fed does not mean organic. Pastured animals sometimes graze on land that has been treated with synthetic fertilizers and even doused with herbicides. Unless the meat label specifically says it is both grass-fed and organic, it isn't.

And then, as seems so often to be the case, there is "green-washing"—a PR effort aimed at misleading the public into thinking a company's policies and products are socially responsible when, in fact, they are not. A case in point is the "premium natural" beef raised by the enormous Harris Ranch located in Fresno County, California. Harris Ranch "premium natural" beef is sold in health food stores west of the Rockies. The company says it is "at the forefront of quality, safety and consumer confidence" with its "premium natural beef."

But even Harris Ranch spokesman Brad Caudill admits that under current USDA rules, the term "natural" is meaningless. Harris Ranch cattle are fattened in a 100,000 cattle feedlot in California's Central Valley. And the feed is not organically grown. The only difference between Harris Ranch "premium natural" beef and the typical feedlot product is that the animals are raised without growth hormones or supplemental antibiotics added to their feed. Despite the marketing and hype, the product is neither organic nor grass-fed. (Harris Ranch also sells a line of organic beef, but the cattle are still raised in over-crowded and filthy feedlots. There can be as many as 100 cattle, weighing from 700 to 1,200 pounds, living in a pen the size of a basketball court.)

THE DARK SIDE

Grass-fed beef certainly has its advantages, but it is typically more expensive, and I'm not at all sure that's a bad thing. We shouldn't be eating nearly as much meat as we do.

And there is a dark side even to grass-fed beef. It takes a lot of grassland to raise a grass-fed steer. Western rangelands are vast, but not nearly vast enough to sustain America's 100 million head of cattle. There is no way that grass-fed beef can begin to feed the current meat appetites of people in the United States, much less play a role in addressing world hunger. Grass-fed meat production may be viable in a country like New Zealand with its geographic isolation, unique climate and topography, and exceedingly small human population. But in a world of 7 billion people, I am afraid that grass-fed beef is a food that only the wealthy elites will be able to consume in any significant quantities.

What would happen if we sought to raise great quantities of grass-fed beef? It's been tried in Brazil and the result has been an environmental nightmare of epic proportions. In 2009, Greenpeace released a report titled "Slaughtering the Amazon," which presented detailed satellite photos showing that Amazon cattle are now the biggest single cause of global deforestation, which is in turn responsible for 20 percent of the world's greenhouse gases. Even Brazil's government, whose policies have made the nation the world's largest beef exporter and home to the planet's largest commercial cattle herd, acknowledges that cattle ranches are responsible for 80 percent of Amazonian deforestation. Much of the remaining 20 percent is for land to grow soy, which is not used to make tofu. It is sold to China to feed livestock.

Amazonian cattle are free-range, grass-fed, and possibly organic, but they are still a plague on the planet and a driving force behind global warming.

Trendy consumers like to think that grass-fed beef is green and Earth-friendly and does not have the environmental problems associated with factory-farmed beef. But grass-fed and feedlot beef production both contribute heavily to global climate change. They do this through emissions of two potent global-warming gases: methane and nitrous oxide.

Next to carbon dioxide, the most destabilizing gas to the planet's climate is methane. Methane is actually twenty-four times more potent a greenhouse gas than carbon dioxide, and its concentration in the atmosphere is rising even faster. The primary reason that concentrations of atmospheric methane are now triple what they were when they began rising a century ago is beef production. Cattle raised on pasture actually produce more methane than feedlot animals, on a per-cow basis. The slower weight gain of a grass-fed animal means that each cow produces methane emissions for a longer time.

Meanwhile, producing a pound of grass-fed beef accounts for every bit as much nitrous oxide emission as producing a pound of feedlot beef, and sometimes, due to the slower weight gain, even more. These emissions are not only fueling global warming. They are also acidifying soils, reducing biodiversity, and shrinking Earth's protective stratospheric ozone layer.

The sobering reality is that cattle-grazing in the U.S. is already taking a tremendous toll on the environment. Even with almost all U.S. beef cattle spending much of their lives in feedlots, 70 percent of the land area of the American West is currently used for grazing livestock. More than two-thirds of the entire land area of Montana, Wyoming, Colorado, New Mexico, Arizona, Nevada, Utah, and Idaho is used for rangeland. In the American West, virtually every place that can be grazed is grazed. The results aren't pretty. As one environmental author put it: "Cattle-grazing in the West has polluted more water, eroded more topsoil, killed more fish, displaced more wildlife, and destroyed more vegetation than any other land use."

Western rangelands have been devastated under the impact of the current system, in which cattle typically spend only about six months on the range, and the rest of their lives in feedlots. To bring cows to market weight on rangeland alone would require each animal to spend not six months foraging, but several years, greatly multiplying the damage to Western ecosystems.

The USDA's taxpayer-funded Animal Damage Control (ADC) program was established in 1931 for a single purpose—to eradicate, suppress, and control wildlife considered detrimental to the Western livestock industry. The program has not been popular with its opponents. They have called the ADC by a variety of names, including, "All the Dead Critters" and "Aid to Dependent Cowboys."

In 1997, following the advice of public relations and image consultants, the federal government gave a new name to the ADC—Wildlife Services. And they came up with a new motto—"Living with Wildlife."

But the agency does not exactly "live with" wildlife. What it actually does is kill any creature that might compete with or threaten livestock. Its methods include poisoning, trapping, snaring, denning, shooting, and aerial gunning. In "denning" wildlife, government agents pour kerosene into the den and then set it on fire, burning the young alive in their nests.

Among the animals Wildlife Services agents intentionally kill are badgers, black bears, bobcats, coyotes, gray fox, red fox, mountain lions, opossum, raccoons, striped skunks, beavers, nutrias, porcupines, prairie dogs, blackbirds, cattle egrets, and starlings. Animals unintentionally killed by Wildlife Services agents include domestic dogs and cats, and several threatened and endangered species.

All told, Wildlife Services intentionally kills more than 1.5 million wild animals annually. This is done at public expense, to protect the private financial interests of ranchers who graze their livestock on public lands, and who pay almost nothing for the privilege.

The price that Western lands and wildlife are paying for grazing cattle is hard to exaggerate. Conscientious management of rangelands can certainly reduce the damage, but widespread production of grass-fed beef would only multiply this already devastating toll. As Edward Abbey, conservationist and author, said in a speech before cattlemen at the University of Montana in 1985:

> Most of the public lands in the West, and especially the Southwest, are what you might call "cow burnt." Almost anywhere and everywhere you go in the American West you find hordes of cows . . . . They are a pest and a plague. They pollute our springs and streams and rivers. They infest our canyons, valleys, meadows and forests. They graze off the native bluestems and grama and bunch grasses, leaving behind jungles of prickly pear. They trample down the native forbs and shrubs and cacti. They spread the exotic cheatgrass, the Russian thistle, and the crested wheat grass. Even when the cattle are not physically present, you see the dung and the flies and the mud and the dust and the general destruction. If you don't see it, you'll smell it. The whole American West stinks of cattle.

Grass-fed beef is certainly much healthier than feedlot beef for the consumer, and may be slightly healthier for the environment. But doing well in such a comparison hardly constitutes a ringing endorsement. While grass-fed beef and other pastured animal products have advantages over factory-farm and feedlot products, it's important to remember that factory-farm and feedlot products are an unmitigated disaster. Almost anything would be an improvement.

I am reminded of a brochure the Cattlemen's Association used to distribute to schools. The pamphlet compared the nutritional realities of a hamburger with another common food, and made much of the fact that the hamburger was superior in that it had more of every single nutrient listed than its competitor. And what's more, the competitor had far more sugar. The comparison made it sound like a hamburger was truly a health food.

The competition, however, was not the stiffest imaginable. It was a 12-ounce can of Coke.

Comparing grass-fed beef to feedlot beef is a little like that. It's far healthier, far more humane, and somewhat more environmentally sustainable, at least on a modest scale. Overall, it's indeed better. If you are going to eat beef, that's the best way to do it.

But I wouldn't get too carried away and think that, as long as it's grass-fed, then the more the better. Grass-fed products are still high in saturated fat (though not as high), still high in cholesterol, and still devoid of fiber and many other essential nutrients. They are still high on the food chain, and often contain elevated concentrations of environmental toxins.

THE SLAUGHTERHOUSE

When you picture grass-fed beef, you probably envision an idyllic scene of a cow outside in a pasture munching happily on grass. That is certainly the image those endorsing and selling these products would like you to hold. And there is some truth to it.

But it is only a part of the story. There is something missing from such a pleasant picture—something that nevertheless remains an ineluctable part of the actual reality. Grass-fed beef does not just come to you straight from God's green Earth. It also comes to you via the slaughterhouse.

The lives of grass-fed livestock are more humane and natural than the lives of animals confined in factory farms and feedlots, but their deaths are often just as terrifying and cruel. If they are taken to a conventional slaughterhouse, as indeed most of them are, they are just as likely as feedlot animals to be skinned while alive and fully conscious, and just as apt to be butchered and have their feet cut off while they are still breathing—distressing realities that tragically occur every hour in meat-packing plants nationwide. Confronting the brutal realities of modern slaughterhouses can be a harsh reminder that those who contemplate only the pastoral image of cattle patiently foraging do not see the whole picture.

IMAGINE

One way to mitigate all these negative impacts is to eat less meat, or even none. If, as a society, we ate meat less, the world would indeed be a brighter and more beautiful place. Consider, for example, the impact on global warming. Gidon Eshel, a geophysicist at the Bard Center, and Pamela A. Martin, Assistant Professor of Geophysics at the University of Chicago, have calculated the benefits that would occur if Americans were to reduce beef consumption by 20 percent. Such a change would decrease our greenhouse gas emissions as substantially as if we exchanged all our cars and trucks for Priuses.

If we ate less meat, the vast majority of the public lands in the western United States could be put to more valuable—and environmentally sustainable—use. Much of the western United States is sunny and windy, and could be used for large-scale solar-energy and wind-power facilities. With the cattle off the land, photovoltaic modules and windmills could generate enormous amounts of energy without polluting or causing environmental damage. Other areas could grow grasses that could be harvested as "biomass" fuels, providing a far less polluting source of energy than fossil fuels. Much of it could be restored, once again becoming valued wildlife habitat. The restoration of cow-burnt lands would help to vitalize our rural economies as well as the planet's ecosystems.

8

Are Factory Farms Becoming Biological Weapons Factories?

ONE OF THE TECHNIQUES modern factory farms routinely use to increase weight in livestock is to give all of the animals a dose of antibiotics with every meal. When this is done, the bacteria in the animals' guts that are susceptible to the drugs are killed.

The problem is that this creates a microbial vacuum in the animals' intestines that gives an extraordinary competitive advantage to any bacteria that develop resistance to the antibiotics. If your goal were to breed bacteria that could not be controlled by antibiotics, you could hardly design a more effective system. It is unfortunately not an exaggeration to say that, as a result, factory farms are unintentionally producing pathogens that may as well be biological weapons.

Antibiotics have saved millions of lives, and their discovery ranks with the great medical achievements of history. But even Sir Alexander Fleming, the man who first discovered penicillin, warned that overuse of the drug would lead to bacterial resistance. And indeed, the drugs have been heavily overused, with increasingly alarming consequences. This year, between 70,000 and 100,000 Americans will die from infections that could once have been cured with common antibiotics. A single antibiotic-resistant pathogen, MRSA (methicillin-resistant *Staphylococcus aureus*), now causes more deaths in the U.S. annually than AIDS.

When it is willing to acknowledge that this problem exists, the livestock industry pins the blame on the overuse of antibiotics in hospitals. And they have a point. The amount of antibiotics used in U.S. hospitals today is hundreds of times greater than it was fifty years ago. As the levels of antibiotic-resistant bacteria have risen, hospitals have tried to cope by using higher doses and employing more antibiotics, particularly the broad-spectrum types. But even with the greatly increased use of these drugs in hospitals, clinics, doctors' offices, and other medical settings, the use of antibiotics in factory farms still accounts for the overwhelming majority of all antibiotic use in the country.

According to the USDA, only about 20 percent of the antibiotics used in the U.S. are administered to people to treat diseases. The other 80 percent—the vast majority—are administered to U.S. livestock, primarily to compensate for the unnatural and unhealthy conditions of factory farming. The result is that industrial livestock systems do not only produce modern meat. They have become factories for the production of resistant bacteria. Of course, this production is not intentional. But that does not reduce its consequences one iota.

Now Congress is considering a bill that would attempt to save the remaining viability of our antibiotics—H.R. 1549, the Preservation of Antibiotics for Medical Treatment Act. Introduced by Representative Louise Slaughter (D-NY), it would prohibit several types of antibiotics from being used routinely in animal feed.

The bill would not ban the use of these medicines to treat sick animals, but rather the practice of routinely administering these drugs to healthy livestock as "growth promotants." Livestock that aren't raised in confinement rarely need antibiotics, but factory farming has grown utterly dependent on the use of the drugs.

Representatives of the modern meat industry argue that if the animals were not routinely fed antibiotics, rates of illness might increase and more antibiotics would be needed to treat the sick animals. But this would occur only if nothing were done to improve the extreme overcrowding, the lack of basic sanitation, and other unhealthy conditions that typify factory farms.

The farm lobby and the drug industry are fighting H.R. 1549, because they know that it would take away a critical support for large-scale intensive-confinement animal agriculture. They want to retain the right to continue the widespread use of the drugs, even though this practice has been proven repeatedly to cause resistance among bacteria, jeopardizing human health and causing diseases that are difficult or impossible to cure.

Dr. Jeffrey Fisher, a pathologist and consultant to the World Health Organization, explains how severe the problem is becoming: "The pendulum has incredibly begun to swing back to the 1930s. Hospitals are in jeopardy of once again being overwhelmed with untreatable infectious diseases such as pneumonia, tuberculosis, meningitis, typhoid fever and dysentery."

How, you may wonder, does the livestock industry manage to defend their current practices? It isn't easy, but they always seem to find a way. If denial were an Olympic sport, their spokesman in recent congressional hearings, Representative John Shimkus (R-IL), might well have earned a gold medal. "So far," he proclaimed, "there's nothing that links use in animals to a buildup of resistance in humans."

I hate to break it to Representative Shimkus, but the scientific consensus that the routine use of antibiotics in animal agriculture is the primary cause of antibiotic-resistant bacteria has been conclusive for many years. Here's a little history lesson for the congressman.

In 1989, the Institute of Medicine, a division of the National Academy of Sciences, stated that the use of antibiotics in factory farms was responsible for antibiotic resistance in bacteria and was seriously undermining the ability of these agents to protect human health. Three years later, the Institute of Medicine stated that multi-drug-resistant bacteria had now become a serious medical concern. The Institute of Medicine laid the problem squarely on the doorstep of Confined Animal Feeding Operations (CAFOs), also known as factory farms.

In 1997, the World Health Organization called for a ban on the routine feeding of antibiotics to livestock. A year later, the journal *Science* called the meat industry "the driving force behind the development of antibiotic resistance in species of bacteria that cause human disease." In 1998, the CDC blamed the serious emergence of salmonella bacteria that had become resistant to no less than five different antibiotics on the routine and non–medically necessary use of antibiotics in livestock.

By then, many nations—including Canada, the United Kingdom, the Netherlands, Sweden, Finland, Denmark, Germany, and many other European countries—had banned the routine feeding of antibiotics to livestock. In the United States, bills have been introduced in Congress repeatedly to follow suit, but lobbying by the meat industry has successfully prevented these bills from becoming law.

Now H.R. 1549 is raising the matter again, and the livestock industry is adamantly opposing the bill. But Pennsylvania Republican Tim Murphy acknowledged that the scientific consensus is becoming incontrovertible. "The vast majority of evidence in the last three decades," he stated in congressional hearings, "points to a linkage between routine, low-level antibiotic use in food animals and the transfer of antibiotic-resistant bacteria to people."

Seventy percent of all healthcare related infections in the U.S. are resistant to at least one antibiotic, Murphy says, which already costs the nation's healthcare system $50 billion a year.

CBS Evening News anchor Katie Couric recently ran a story on the topic, reporting: "This week on Capitol Hill, critics are worried that giving antibiotics to livestock, unless medically necessary, may be creating dangerous, drug-resistant bacteria that can be passed on to humans."

The livestock industry, as you may imagine, was not pleased with Ms. Couric.

"Oh Katie, were you ever really a journalist or always just a wannabe?" huffed a spokesman for the beef industry. He called her report a "witch hunt" that was biased "against the concept of healthy farm animals."

But when it comes to denial, you really do have to hand it to the National Cattlemen's Beef Association. Unperturbed by something as minor as the conclusions of nearly every public health expert and public health organization in the world, the organization tells us that "antibiotic use in animal agriculture makes a very small contribution to the resistance issue."

Very small? Not according to Dr. Frederick J. Angulo, an epidemiologist at the Centers for Disease Control and Prevention. "Public health is united in the conclusion," he says. "There is no controversy about where antibiotic resistance in food-borne pathogens comes from. It is due to the heavy use of antibiotics in livestock."

The influence of the modern meat industry is so strong, however, that H.R. 1549 is unlikely to become law, and may not even make it out of committee. This is a shame. Dr. Ali Khan, Deputy Director of the CDC, told Congress in 2011 that the evidence implicating the use of antibiotics in animal agriculture in the creation of antibiotic-resistant bacteria is "unequivocal and compelling."

Without legislation, we are left with the FDA "urging" the industry to limit their use of antibiotics voluntarily. But producers aren't going to hold back on using the drugs if they think doing so will put them at a competitive disadvantage compared with other producers who continue to use them. Meanwhile, bacteria are continuing to develop resistance, and we are becoming increasingly vulnerable to life-threatening diseases that we can no longer treat successfully.

The widespread use of antibiotics in animal agriculture does faintly increase the yield and profit margin obtained by factory farms. But do the American people really think that slightly enhancing the profitability of factory farming is more important than the future viability of what are certainly among the most significant medical tools ever developed?

9

Greed and Salmonella:
A Deadly Duo

FOR YEARS, THE U.S. EGG INDUSTRY has been telling us that there is no connection between salmonella outbreaks and the practice of cramming layer hens into cages so small the birds can't lift a wing. It's been their party line for so long they've actually probably begun to believe it. In 2011, the leading U.S. egg industry trade group announced, true to form, that caging hens is "better for food safety."

With more than 95 percent of all U.S. eggs currently coming from caged hens, and salmonella outbreaks sickening more than one million Americans every year, this isn't merely an academic debate. Salmonella poisons people, causing a nasty, painful disease that can be fatal to the very young, the elderly, and anyone with a weakened immune system.

As you've probably heard, we have been experiencing a string of salmonella outbreaks caused by bad eggs. More than 500 million eggs were recently recalled in one two-week period. And once again, industry representatives are claiming the problem has nothing to do with the practice of housing hens for their entire lives in cages where they are barely able to move. Anyone who tells you otherwise, they say, is probably an animal rights zealot with a hidden agenda.

But wait a minute. The editor-in-chief of the trade journal *Egg Industry* is certainly not what most people would call an animal rights advocate. What is his opinion of the industry position that squishing living birds into tiny cages has no bearing on public health? Such claims, he wrote recently, not mincing his words, are "invalid . . . unconvincing, unsupportable and easily refuted."

Though his remarks may not be popular at the next gathering of egg industry moguls, they are, in fact, correct. There have been nine scientific studies published on the issue in the last five years in peer-reviewed journals. Every single one of them has found increased salmonella rates in eggs coming from facilities that confine hens in cages.

A 2010 article in *World Poultry*, aptly titled "Salmonella Thrives in Cage Housing," found that eggs from hens kept in cages consistently carry an increased risk of salmonella.

The Humane Society of the United States (HSUS) recently began an ad campaign pointing out that every one of the more than half a billion eggs involved in a recent large-scale recall came from hens crammed into cages. The practice of forcing egg-laying hens to live their entire lives in tiny cages isn't just an animal welfare concern, say the ads. It is a public health issue. Housing hens in cages so small they can't take a single step is not just inhumane. It's a public health menace.

Should we be suspicious of the HSUS? The group is, of course, fundamentally an animal protection organization. But does that automatically mean they are stretching the truth? Not according to a study published in *The American Journal of Epidemiology*. The study suggests that by switching to cage-free production systems, the egg industry could likely reduce the risk of salmonella to the American public from bad eggs by 50 percent.

How do you think the egg industry is taking all this? Are they afraid of being held financially accountable for the damage to human health caused by their tainted products? Not really, for they rest secure in the knowledge that America's food-safety systems have been designed, not to protect public health, but to protect agribusiness from liability.

So why rock the boat?

Except that the boat is already rocking. As of January 2012, it became illegal to house laying hens in cages anywhere in the European Union. In the U.S., the states of Michigan and California have already passed laws phasing out the practice of confining hens in cages. In California, Governor Arnold Schwarzenegger has signed a bill requiring that all whole eggs sold in the state be cage-free by 2015. And other states are considering similar legislation.

The egg industry defends the status quo by threatening that healthier eggs from better-treated birds would be vastly more expensive, and thus would mean more malnutrition among the poor. It's a powerful argument, except it's not true. If you factor in the economies of scale, going cage-free need add only about a penny per egg to the retail price.

This is why a number of major fast-food companies, including Burger King, Subway, and Wendy's, and retailers including Trader Joe's, Safeway, and Walmart, have made various levels of commitment to purchasing or selling cage-free eggs. And why major food companies like Hellmann's (called Best Foods in Western states), which uses 350 million eggs a year in its mayonnaise, have announced they are going 100 percent cage-free.

McDonald's in the U.S. has been a little slower to get the message. One of the burger giant's executives recently said he didn't think hens "should be treated like queens." But does going "cage-free" mean the hens will be treated like royalty? Far from it. Cage-free does not mean cruelty-free. But at least cage-free hens will have two to three times more space per bird than caged hens. And unlike caged hens, they will be able to stand up, fully extend their limbs, lie down, and turn around.

From an animal welfare point of view, cage-free eggs are far from perfect, but they are better. And from a public health perspective, cage-free eggs are a necessary and urgently needed improvement.

What can you do?

- Take the HSUS "cage-free pledge."

- If you are going to eat eggs, seek out organic and free-range eggs.

- Never eat raw eggs.

- Don't spend extra for brown eggs. They aren't any more nutritious than white eggs; they are just from a different breed of hens.

- Don't be fooled by eggs that claim they are produced without added hormones. That sounds nice, but is meaningless. No hormones are currently approved for use in U.S. egg production.

- Be aware that the egg industry has been eager to co-opt the language of humane farming. As awareness of the horrors of egg factory farms has been growing in recent years, the industry trade group United Egg Producers responded, not by improving conditions, but by labeling cartons of eggs "Animal Care Certified." In actuality, this "certification" was only the industry's misleading attempt to whitewash its tarnished image. After legal action forced them to remove the meaningless label, the industry came up with yet another bogus attempt to hoodwink the public. Egg cartons that say "Produced in Compliance with United Egg Producers Animal Husbandry Guidelines" are designed to help you feel safe and confident as you purchase eggs that come from filthy disease mills, including the very facilities whose salmonella-infected eggs are the target of the recent spate of recalls.

- If you are going to eat eggs, try to bypass the supermarket entirely and get them from local farmers' markets. To find one near you, go to *www.localharvest.org*.

At the moment, cage-free, free-range, and organic eggs are indeed more expensive. Are they worth the added cost? That's up to the buyer to decide. But the more you learn, the more able you are to make informed choices. When you include the risk of salmonella poisoning, when you take into account the differences in flavor and nutrition, and when you factor in the degree of animal cruelty involved, getting away from eggs that come from concentration-camp chickens starts to seem less like a luxury. The more you know, the more it seems like an ethical and health imperative.

10

Infants Growing Breasts: The Trouble with Hormones in Our Milk

FEMALE INFANTS IN CHINA who have been fed formula have been growing breasts. People are very upset about this, and for good reason.

According to the official Chinese daily newspaper, medical tests performed on the babies between four and fifteen months old found levels of estrogen circulating in their bloodstreams that are as high as those found in most adult women. The milk formula they have been fed appears to be responsible.

Synutra, the company that makes the baby formula consumed by these babies, says it's not their fault. They insist that "no man-made hormones or any illegal substances were added during the production of the milk powder."

Then what is the source of the hormones? A Chinese dairy association says the hormones could have entered the food chain when farmers reared the cows. "Since a regulation forbidding the use of hormones to cultivate livestock has yet to be drawn up in China," says Wang Dingmian, former chairman of the dairy association in the southern province of Guangdo, "it would be lying to say nobody uses it." Bovine growth hormones are used in China, as they are in the U.S., to promote greater milk production.

An extraordinary number of food products sold in the U.S. today come from China. Could some of this tainted formula be making its way to the U.S.?

There is currently no way for consumers to know whether infant formula they purchase has been made with milk products from China.

If this problem appears in the U.S., who will be held responsible? The retailers? The importers? The Chinese producers? Will anyone be called to account?

This isn't the first time something like this has happened. In the 1980s, doctors in Puerto Rico began encountering cases of precocious puberty—four-year-old girls with fully developed breasts; three-year-old girls with pubic hair and vaginal bleeding; one-year-old girls who had not yet begun to walk, but whose breasts were growing. And it wasn't just the females. Young boys were also affected. Many had to have surgery to deal with breasts that had become grossly swollen.

Writing a few years later in *The Journal of the Puerto Rico Medical Association*, Dr. Carmen A. Saenz explained the cause: "It was clearly observed in 97 percent of the cases that the appearance of abnormal breast tissue was . . . related to local whole milk in the infants."

The problem was traced to, and found to stem from, the misuse of hormones in dairy cows. When Dr. Saenz was asked how she could be certain the babies and children were contaminated with hormones from milk rather than from some other source, she replied simply: "When we take our young patients off . . . fresh milk, their symptoms usually regress."

Along with China, the U.S. is today one of the few countries in the world that still allows bovine growth hormones to be injected into dairy cows. Though banned in Canada,

Japan, Australia, New Zealand, and most of Europe, the use of these hormones in U.S. dairy is not only legal; it's routine in all fifty states.

The U.S. dairy industry assures us that this is not a problem. But there is a very real problem, and its name is Insulin-like Growth Factor-1 (IGF-1). Monsanto's own studies, as well as those of Eli Lilly & Co., have found an up to ten-fold increase in IGF-1 levels in the milk of cows that have been injected with bovine growth hormone (BGH).

Why is this a problem? A report by the European Commission's authoritative sixteen-member international scientific committee confirmed that excessive levels of IGF-1 are always found in the milk of cows injected with BGH. It also concluded that excess levels of IGF-1 may pose serious risks of breast, colon, and prostate cancer.

How serious is the increased risk? According to an article in the May 9, 1998 issue of the medical journal *Lancet*, women with even a relatively small increase in blood levels of IGF-1 are up to seven times more likely to develop breast cancer than women with lower levels.

IGF-1 that is consumed by human beings in dairy products is rapidly absorbed into the bloodstream. It isn't destroyed by human digestion. And pasteurization is no help. In fact, the pasteurization process actually increases IGF-1 levels in milk.

What's a consumer to do?

If at all possible, breast-feed your babies, and support breastfeeding-friendly workplaces and other environments. It's hard to overstate the health advantages of breastfeeding for both mother and baby. They are enormous, and particularly so today, when the possibility exists that commercially available infant formula could be contaminated with excess hormones.

If you are going to buy dairy products, try to get them from organic sources. Organic milk products, by law, can't be produced with bovine growth hormone (BGH). Or look for dairy products that specifically say they are produced without BGH (also called recombinant bovine somatotropin, or rBST). Starbucks uses only dairy products that have not been produced with the hormone. Ben & Jerry's ice cream likewise uses only milk and cream from dairy farms that have pledged not to use BGH.

If you're going to eat cheese, remember that American-made cheeses are likely to be contaminated with BGH and excess levels of IGF-1 unless they're organic or labeled BGH-free. Most cheeses that are imported from Europe are safe, however, since much of Europe has banned the hormone.

Have you ever wondered why dairy products made from cows injected with the hormone aren't labeled? It's because Monsanto, the original manufacturer of BGH, has aggressively and successfully lobbied state governments to make sure that no legislation is passed that would require such labeling.

As if that weren't enough, Monsanto has also insistently sought to make it illegal for dairy products that are BGH-free to say so on their labels, unless the labels also include wording exonerating BGH. How does Monsanto justify such a ban? They say that allowing retailers to tell consumers that a dairy product is BGH-free shouldn't be allowed, even if it's true, because it unfairly stigmatizes BGH.

Monsanto acts as if accurately labeling products makes them the victim of some irrational cultural bias. But the company's products are, in fact, responsible for untold damage to human health.

11

Is Your Favorite Ice Cream Made with Monsanto's Artificial Hormones?

MONSANTO HAS BEEN IN THE NEWS again, with a U.S. District Court ruling that the USDA has to at least go through the motions of regulating the company's genetically engineered sugar beets. Monsanto, you may know, is not likely to win any contests for the most popular company. In fact, it has been called the most hated corporation in the world—which is saying something, given the competition from the likes of BP, Halliburton, and Goldman Sachs.

This has gotten me thinking about, of all things, ice cream, and of how Monsanto's clammy paws can be found in some of the most widely sold ice cream brands in the country. These brands could break free from Monsanto's clutches. So far they haven't, but maybe this is about to change.

Ben & Jerry's gets all their milk from dairies that have pledged not to inject their cows with genetically engineered bovine growth hormone (rBGH). Why, then, can't Häagen-Dazs, Breyers, and Baskin-Robbins do the same?

Starbucks now guarantees that all their milk, cream, and other dairy products are rBGH-free. So do Yoplait and Dannon yogurts, Tillamook cheese, Chipotle restaurants, and many others. But ice cream giants Häagen-Dazs, Breyers, and Baskin-Robbins continue to use milk from cows injected with rBGH, a hormone that's been banned in Canada, New Zealand, Japan, Australia, and all twenty-seven nations of the European Union. As if to add insult to injury, Häagen-Dazs and Breyers have the audacity to tell us, right on the label, that their ice cream is "All Natural."

We have Monsanto to thank for rBGH. Monsanto developed the artificial hormone and marketed it aggressively for years before selling it in 2008 to Elanco, a division of the Eli Lilly drug company. Of course, Monsanto (and now Elanco) wants us to think the hormone is in every way completely satisfactory and safe. Monsanto's party line has consistently been that there is "no significant difference" in the milk derived from cows who have been dosed with the hormone compared with those who haven't.

Pardon me for not swallowing Monsanto's hooey, but if that's so, why have so many countries outlawed rBGH? Are these countries all run by ignorant Luddites who oppose technology and progress? Or could there actually be compelling reasons?

There are, indeed. One of them is that injecting the genetically engineered hormone into cows increases the levels of IGF-1 in their milk. Monsanto's own studies found that the amount of IGF-1 in milk more than doubled when cows were injected with rBGH. Studies by independent researchers show increases as high as ten-fold, which seriously increases the risk of many forms of cancer. Women with elevated levels of IGF-1 are up to seven times more likely to develop breast cancer.

As if these risks to human health weren't enough reason for nations to prohibit the use of rBGH, there are more. The artificial hormone is also notorious for causing the cows much pain and distress. It does this by increasing painful and debilitating diseases like lameness and mastitis in cows that are injected with it. And because it increases udder infections in cows, it has greatly increased the use of antibiotics in the U.S. dairy industry.

Does the increase in udder infections have an effect on the milk, and thus any ice cream, cheese, or other product made from it? Most definitely, according to Dr. Richard Burroughs, a veterinarian deeply familiar with rBGH. "It results in an increase of white blood cells," he says, "which means there's pus in the milk!" The antibiotic use, he adds, "leaves residues in the milk. It's all very serious."

How, then, was such a dubious and tainted product ever approved for use in the U.S.? The answer provides a glimpse into how successful Monsanto's efforts have been to exert control over our nation's food policies.

By all accounts, the FDA's 1993 decision to allow the use of rBGH was one of the most controversial in the agency's history. Made amid widespread criticism from scientists, government leaders, and farmers—including many researchers and officials inside the FDA—the decision was overseen by Michael R. Taylor, the FDA's Deputy Commissioner of Policy from 1991 to 1994.

Was Taylor unbiased? Prior to holding his position at the FDA, he was an attorney at King & Spaulding, Monsanto's law firm, where he presided over the firm's food-and-drug law practice. After the decision was made that gave the green light to rBGH, he left the FDA and resumed working directly for Monsanto, as vice president and chief lobbyist.

How significant was Taylor's role in getting rBGH approved? On August 15, 2010, his Wikipedia entry said that he "has long been hostile to food safety," and "is widely credited with ushering recombinant bovine growth hormone (rBGH) through the FDA regulatory process and into the milk supply—unlabeled." (This statement was removed from Wikipedia immediately after I referred to it in a comment following an article I wrote for *Huffington Post* on the topic. Apparently, if you can get your people in and out of key positions at the FDA, messing with Wikipedia is a piece of cake.)

Congressman Bernie Sanders was probably referring to Taylor when he said "the FDA allowed corporate influence to run rampant in its approval of rBGH." Documentaries including *The World According to Monsanto* and *The Future of Food* present Taylor's pro-Monsanto actions at the FDA as a dramatic example of how corporate influence has exerted massive control over the agency. Today, Taylor again works for the FDA, now as Deputy Commissioner of Foods.

Things have taken a different turn in Canada, but not for want of effort on the part of Monsanto. During Canada's scientific review of Monsanto's application for approval of rBGH, Canadian health officials said Monsanto tried to bribe them, and government scientists testified that they were being pressured by higher-ups to approve rBGH against their better scientific judgment. But in 1999, after eight years of study, Canadian health authorities rejected Monsanto's application for approval of rBGH.

In the U.S. today, Monsanto continues to wield massive influence over national food policies. In spite of, or perhaps in response to, Monsanto's toxic and tenacious grip on our nation's food policy, a movement is afoot. Every day more and more people are refusing to buy ice cream and other dairy products made with rBGH. And every day another organization adds its name to the growing list of groups campaigning against Monsanto's influence, and calling for the FDA decision allowing the use of rBGH to be revoked.

Late last year, the prestigious American Public Health Association officially called for a ban on rBGH. The Consumers Union, publishers of *Consumer Reports*, has likewise taken an official position opposing rBGH. So has the American Nurses Association, Health Care without Harm, Food and Water Watch, the Center for Food Safety, National Family Farm Coalition, Family Farm Defenders, and many other groups.

At this very moment, the plucky Oregon chapter of Physicians for Social Responsibility (PSR) is leading a nationwide effort to persuade Breyers (whose brands include Good Humor, Klondike Bars, and Popsicle), and Dreyer's (whose brands include Häagen-Dazs, Nestlé, and Edy's) to go rBGH-free. The campaign focuses on Breyers and Dreyer's because they are the two largest ice cream producers in the country today.

Monsanto and its allies have a grand vision. They are intent on controlling the world's food supply. Don't let them. And don't let them cram their genetically engineered products down your throat. Even in a product as tempting and sweet as ice cream, that's no treat.

12

The Startling Health Benefits
of Dark Chocolate

THE FOOD POLICE MAY FIND THIS HARD to take, but chocolate has gotten a bad rap. People say it causes acne, that you should eat carob instead, that it's junk food. But these accusations are not only undeserved and inaccurate; they falsely incriminate a delicious food that turns out to have profoundly important healing powers.

There is, in fact, a growing body of credible scientific evidence that chocolate contains a host of heart-healthy and mood-enhancing phytochemicals that are beneficial to both body and mind.

For one, chocolate is a plentiful source of antioxidants. These are substances that reduce the ongoing cellular and arterial damage caused by oxidative reactions.

You may have heard of a type of antioxidants called polyphenols. These are protective chemicals found in plant foods like red wine and green tea. Chocolate, it turns out, is particularly rich in polyphenols. According to researchers at the University of Texas Southwestern Medical Center in Dallas, the same antioxidant properties found in red wine that protect against heart disease are also found in comparable quantities in chocolate.

How does chocolate help to prevent heart disease? The oxidation of LDL cholesterol is considered a major factor in the promotion of coronary disease. When this waxy substance oxidizes, it tends to stick to artery walls, increasing the risk of a heart attack or stroke. But chocolate to the rescue! The polyphenols in chocolate inhibit oxidation of LDL cholesterol.

And there's more. One of the causes of atherosclerosis is blood platelets clumping together, a process called aggregation. The polyphenols in chocolate inhibit this clumping, reducing the risk of atherosclerosis.

High blood pressure is a well-known risk factor for heart disease. It is also one of the most common causes of kidney failure, and a significant contributor to many kinds of dementia and cognitive impairment. Studies have shown that consuming a small bar of dark chocolate daily can reduce blood pressure in people with mild hypertension.

Why are people with risk factors for heart disease sometimes told to take a baby aspirin every day? The reason is that aspirin thins the blood and reduces the likelihood of clots forming (clots play a key role in many heart attacks and strokes). Research performed at the Department of Nutrition at the University of California Davis found that chocolate thins the blood and performs the same anti-clotting activity as aspirin. "Our work supports the concept that the chronic consumption of cocoa may be associated with improved cardiovascular health," said UC Davis researcher Carl Keen.

How much chocolate should you eat to obtain these benefits? Less than you may think. According to a study published in the *American Journal of Clinical Nutrition*, adding only half an ounce of dark chocolate to the average daily American diet is enough to increase total antioxidant capacity by 4 percent, and lessen oxidation of LDL cholesterol.

Why, then, has chocolate gotten such a bum reputation? It's the ingredients we add to it. Nearly all of the calories in a typical chocolate bar are sugar and fat.

As far as fats go, it's the added fats that are the difficulty, not the natural fat (called cocoa butter) found in chocolate. Cocoa butter is high in saturated fat, so many people assume that it's not good for your cardiovascular system. But most of the saturated fat content in cocoa butter is stearic acid, which numerous studies have shown does not raise blood cholesterol levels. In the human body, it acts much like the mono-unsaturated fat in olive oil.

Milk chocolate, on the other hand, contains added butterfat that can raise blood cholesterol levels. And it has fewer antioxidants and other beneficial phytochemicals than dark chocolate.

Does chocolate contribute to acne? Milk chocolate has been shown to do so, but I've never heard of any evidence incriminating dark chocolate in that regard.

Dark chocolate is also healthier because it has less added sugar. I'm sure you don't need another lecture on the dangers of excess sugar consumption. But if you want to become obese and dramatically raise your odds of developing diabetes, heart disease, cancer, and Alzheimer's disease, foods high in sugar (including high-fructose corn syrup) are just the ticket.

Are chocolate's benefits limited to the health of the body? Hardly. Chocolate has long been known for its remarkable effects on human mood. We are now beginning to understand why.

Chocolate is the richest known source of a little-known substance called theobromine, a close chemical relative of caffeine. Theobromine, like caffeine, and also like the asthma drug theophylline, belongs to the chemical group known as xanthine alkaloids. Chocolate products contain small amounts of caffeine, but not nearly enough to explain the attractions, fascinations, addictions, and effects of chocolate. The mood enhancement produced by chocolate may be primarily due to theobromine.

Chocolate also contains other substances with mood-elevating effects. One is phenethylamine, which triggers the release of pleasurable endorphins and potentiates the action of dopamine, a neurochemical associated with sexual arousal and pleasure. Phenethylamine is released in the brain when people become infatuated or fall in love.

Another substance found in chocolate is anandamide (from the Sanskrit word *ananda*, which means "peaceful bliss"). A fatty substance that is naturally produced in the brain, anandamide has been isolated from chocolate by pharmacologists at the Neurosciences Institute in San Diego. It binds to the same receptor sites in the brain as cannabinoids—the psychoactive constituents in marijuana—and produces feelings of elation and exhilaration. (If this becomes more widely known, will chocolate be made illegal?)

If that weren't enough, chocolate also boosts brain levels of serotonin. Women typically have lower serotonin levels during PMS and menstruation, which may be one reason why women typically experience stronger cravings for chocolate at these times in their cycles. People suffering from depression are also characteristically known to have lower serotonin levels, to the extent that an entire class of anti-depressive medications called selective serotonin reuptake inhibitors, or SSRIs (including Prozac, Paxil, and Zoloft), have been developed to raise brain levels of serotonin.

Since I am known as an advocate of healthy eating, I'm often asked about my food indulgences. One of my favorite desserts is a piece of dark organic chocolate, along with a glass of a fine red wine.

I do have a policy, however, to eat only organic and/or fair trade chocolate. This is because of what I have learned about child slavery in the cocoa trade, a topic to which we will now turn.

May your life be full of healthy pleasures.

PART THREE

Industrial Food Production— and Other Dirty Dealings

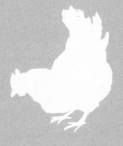

13

No Sweetness Here: Chocolate and 21st-Century Slavery

CHOCOLATE, AS WE'VE JUST SEEN, has extraordinary health benefits. And as just about everyone knows, it's yummy. The very word conjures feelings of pleasure, sensuality, and the richness of life. Is it entirely a surprise that the scientific name of the tree from whose beans we make chocolate, *Theobroma cacao*, literally translates as "food of the gods"?

In some cultures, chocolate has been placed even above gold in value. When Cortez and his Conquistadors first encountered the Aztecs, they were amazed to find a thriving metropolis with more than one million residents, making it several times larger than the biggest city in Europe at the time. Cortez and his band were confronting a culture and an ecosystem that was wildly strange to them. Yet what they found most astonishing was the fact that the royal coffers were overflowing, not with gold, but with cocoa beans. Here, gold was used primarily for architectural and artistic ornament and had only secondary monetary value. The coin of the realm in pre-conquest Mexico was not gold; it was cocoa beans. When Cortez arrived in the Aztec capital, the royal coffers held more than 9,000 tons of cocoa beans.

Since these beans were money, they were roasted and eaten only by the wealthiest citizens. According to the reports of the

Conquistadors, the Aztec emperor drank only cocoa potions. This may have been one of the most extreme examples of conspicuous consumption in history—the eating of money itself.

The Aztec emperor encountered by Cortez and his men is known to popular history as Montezuma II. At the height of his power, this emperor had a stash of a billion cocoa beans, all extracted brutally through the hard labor of his subjects.

Historians say that Montezuma was as feared and hated as any man who ever lived. Notorious for his cruelty and rapaciousness, and infamous for his depravity and decadence, he routinely presided over the sacrificing of human beings to "guarantee" a good cocoa harvest.

Although in our times, we tend to think of chocolate as a sensual treat that almost anyone can afford, down through history chocolate has been a luxury consumed by the privileged at the cost of those much less fortunate. For thousands of years, writes investigative journalist Carol Off in her book *Bitter Chocolate: The Dark Side of the World's Most Seductive Sweet*, the chocolate cravings of an elite have been satisfied by the hard labor of an underclass.

THE DARKNESS TODAY

Tragically, this dark side of chocolate does, in fact, continue today. Most Americans are still unaware of it, but the bleak underbelly of chocolate production was brought to the consciousness of the American public in May 2001, when the Knight Ridder newspapers across the country ran a series of investigative articles about chocolate production. The articles revealed that the chocolate we so love to consume was often being made by child slaves.

In riveting detail, the series profiled young boys who were tricked into slavery, or sold as slaves to Ivory Coast cocoa farmers. Ivory Coast, located on the southern coast of West Africa, is by far the world's largest producer of cocoa beans, providing 43 percent of the world's supply. There are 600,000 cocoa farms in Ivory Coast. Together they account for one-third of the nation's entire economy.

A concurrent investigative report by the British Broadcasting Company (BBC) indicated the size of the problem. According to the BBC, hundreds of thousands of children were being purchased from their parents for a pittance—or in some cases stolen outright—and then shipped to Ivory Coast where they were sold as slaves to cocoa farms.

These children typically came from countries like Mali, Burkina Faso, and Togo. Destitute parents in these poverty-stricken lands were selling their children to traffickers believing that they would find honest work once they arrived in Ivory Coast and then send some of their earnings home. But that's not what was happening. These children—usually eleven to sixteen years old, but sometimes younger—were being forced to do hard manual labor 80 to 100 hours a week. They were paid nothing, were barely fed, were beaten regularly, and were often viciously punished if they tried to escape. Most would never see their families again.

"The beatings were a part of my life," Aly Diabate, a freed slave, told reporters. "Any time they loaded you with bags [of cocoa beans] and you fell while carrying them, nobody helped you. Instead they beat you and beat you until you picked it up again."

Brian Woods and Kate Blewett made a film about the use of child slaves in African cocoa fields. "We literally walked onto plantations and found slave after slave after slave," the film-makers explained in an interview. They met boys who told them they had not been paid a cent even after a year's work. The young people described beatings, starvation diets, and filthy living conditions. Their backs were lacerated from repeated whippings.

Blewett and Woods tell of meeting Drissa, a young man from Mali who had been tricked into working on an Ivory

Coast cocoa farm. "When Drissa took his shirt off, I had never seen anything like it. I had seen some pretty nasty things in my time but this was appalling. There wasn't an inch of his body that wasn't scarred."

PRESSURE FOR CHANGE

Chocolate is a symbol of sweetness and innocence, but Western chocolate consumers know there is nothing sweet and nothing innocent about enslaving children. As publicity about the use of child slaves in the chocolate industry mounted throughout the summer of 2001, so did pressure on the chocolate manufacturers.

That July, Congressman Eliot Engel, representing New York's 17th district, attached a rider to a routine agricultural appropriations bill proposing a labeling system that would certify chocolate products to be "slave free" if it could be documented that the chocolate didn't stem from the work of exploited children. "It would be like the certification on cans of tuna that say 'dolphin safe,'" Engel explained.

The big players in the U.S. chocolate industry were not at all pleased with this turn of events. The two largest U.S. chocolate companies, Mars and Hershey, immediately sent representatives to meet with Congressman Engel. "Their attitude surprised me," Engel said after the meeting. "They were hostile and belligerent. It was all about the bottom line."

Knowing that, by even the most minimal standards, their products could not qualify as "slave-free," the largest chocolate companies fought hard against the impending legislation. Susan Smith, the vice president of public affairs for the Chocolate Manufacturers Association (CMA), questioned whether children were actually being exploited in chocolate production. "A lot of us grew up on farms," she said, "and we know it's normal for children to work." Other public relations professionals employed by the chocolate industry implied that these were just kids being asked to help out on farms, to do their chores, and that the real exploitation was being perpetrated by news organizations who were manufacturing sensational stories. Big Chocolate repeatedly urged legislators not to be misled by "the hearsay reports of overexcited journalists."

Desperate to ward off any kind of labeling, the industry came up with another argument, apparently not noticing that it contradicted the first one. "A 'slave free' label would hurt the people it is intended to help," said CMA vice president Smith, because it would lead to a boycott of all Ivory Coast cocoa. No company using Ivory Coast cocoa could possibly state that none of its chocolate was produced by child slavery, she said, because slave-picked beans were mixed with others harvested by free field hands.

On the one hand, the industry was saying that labeling was a bad idea because child slavery was just a figment of overheated journalists' imaginations. On the other, it was saying that it was a bad idea because child slaves were used so routinely in Ivory Coast cocoa production that the only way to avoid it was to boycott the nation that was producing nearly half of the world's chocolate supply.

The World Cocoa Foundation, Big Chocolate's philanthropic front, commissioned its own study. Not surprisingly, the report ended up claiming that the degree of child exploitation was being exaggerated. Cocoa farmers, according to the study, were simply following standard business practices by employing the cheapest possible labor to harvest and process their beans.

But if the report authorized and paid for by the World Cocoa Foundation was intended to take Big Chocolate off the hook, it did not entirely succeed. For even the industry's own study, designed though it was to minimize the problem, acknowledged that hundreds of thousands of children were working in hazardous conditions on cocoa farms in West Africa, and that these children were living in abject poverty, receiving no schooling or medical care and no pay for their labor. It confirmed that they were subject to brutality if they disobeyed, and that many had been placed in their "jobs" by child traffickers.

Pressure on the industry mounted. By fall 2001, the legislation to adopt "slave-free" labels on chocolate products had passed the House of Representatives (where it was sponsored by Representative Eliot Engel) and was certain to pass in the Senate (where it was sponsored by Senator Tom Harkin).

Concerned to avert labeling, the chocolate industry declared itself committed to a four-year plan that it claimed would eventually eliminate child slavery in cocoa-producing nations, and particularly in West Africa where most of the world's chocolate is grown. If all went according to the plan, the so-called Harkin-Engel Protocol, it would ensure that the "worst forms of child labor"—including slavery—would no longer be used to produce chocolate and cocoa by 2005. The agreement was signed by the World Cocoa Foundation, as well as chocolate producers Hershey, M&M Mars, Nestlé, and many others.

A deal was made. The Harkin-Engel Protocol was announced triumphantly to the world and the legislation was withdrawn. The chocolate industry managed to talk Congress into a voluntary agreement in place of legislation that would have created a mandatory slave-free label for chocolate.

A greatly relieved Larry Graham, president of the Chocolate Manufacturers' Association, promised that "the industry has changed, permanently and forever." A series of deadlines was part of the plan. Industry-wide voluntary standards of public certification were to be in place by July 1, 2005.

Four years later, however, on February 14, 2005, Representative Engel and Senator Harkin co-wrote an op-ed piece that appeared in major U.S. newspapers condemning the chocolate companies for a nearly complete failure to adhere to the agreement. What the industry had done in the intervening four years, said the congressmen, "falls woefully short of the action promised in the protocol. . . . This Valentine's Day, much of our chocolate will be tainted by the suffering of countless cocoa slaves."

The industry immediately issued statements justifying the delay and extolling how much progress had been made. Vowing to "redouble" their efforts, they promised to meet a new deadline in 2008.

At this point the World Cocoa Foundation proudly announced that the industry was voluntarily donating $6 million in "partnerships" to aid agencies. The aid agencies themselves, however, pointed out that the chocolate companies wanted something in return for these "partnerships"— to purloin the good names of the aid agencies as evidence they were doing something meaningful about the problem.

A Hershey representative called one journalist "a cynical party-pooper" for mentioning that spending $6 million in an effort to buy the appearance of virtue was not overly impressive from an industry that was netting upward of $13 billion in annual profits.

Industry spokespeople guaranteed that, by the new deadline of 2008, the problem would be resolved. But when the 2008 deadline rolled around, not a single one of the key promises of the Protocol had been met. And what had happened to the "standards of public certification" that were to be in place by July 1, 2005? Not only were they not in place three years later, but the industry was taking itself off the hook by referring to its former promises as a certification "concept."

Adrienne Fitch-Frankel, the Fair Trade Director of Global Exchange, a national human rights organization based in San Francisco, commented:

> Wouldn't it be great if we could all be released from our moral and legal responsibilities by redefining them? We

can hear the chuckles . . . forming around water coolers nationwide already. Think a repayment "concept" will work for my mortgage? Will the boss buy into a punctuality "concept"?

Spokespeople for Big Chocolate were now blaming the industry's failure on a war that had broken out in Ivory Coast, but journalists familiar with the situation pointed out that the industry's initiatives to deal with the abuse had all along amounted to nothing more than window dressing.

Meanwhile, the exploitation of children on the cocoa farms of Ivory Coast continues.

HERSHEY, NOW AND THEN

We live in cynical times. We are no longer surprised when we find that a major company like BP or Monsanto has done something horrible, and then compounded the damage by hiding the consequences of its actions from the public. We have become used to industries covering up their abuses of human rights and the environment.

But even in a day of such widespread abuse of power, there is a tragic and painful irony to the operations of the nation's second-largest chocolate purveyor, the Hershey Company. Milton Hershey, the company's founder, was a humanitarian and an idealist who was inspired by a Utopian vision. He wanted to create a society where, in his words, there would be "no poverty and no evil."

It was at the dawn of the 20th century that Milton Hershey began to build what would become the city of Hershey, Pennsylvania. Using the proceeds from his candy factory, and determined to create a town of his own, he undertook a daring social experiment. The community he created was unlike anything in America at the time. The streets were broad and tree-lined, and every house had expansive green lawns, indoor plumbing, electricity, and steam heat. These were luxuries most American factory workers, accustomed to coal lamps and outhouses, could barely imagine. And all of this was available to every worker at the Hershey factory at affordable rents, or through low-interest mortgages from the Hershey Trust Bank.

The centerpiece of the town was the chocolate factory, but it also featured a lake-sized swimming pool, a community center with an enormous theater, a bandstand, a golf course, acres of community gardens, and a vast network of public transportation via trolley lines. Every employee enjoyed insurance benefits, healthcare, and a retirement plan.

The tycoons of capitalism were shocked. They called Hershey's enterprise immoral, saying that such generosity "saps a community's self-reliance and injures its pride."

But Milton Hershey was undeterred, and remained dedicated to his Utopian vision. When he and his wife, Catherine, realized that they were unable to bear children, they established an orphanage and took in homeless children. At the time, most of the nation's orphanages were bleak and depressing institutions. But the children taken in by the Hershey orphanage were not only given an education, they lived in the homes of the company's employees.

When Milton Hershey died in 1945, the primary beneficiary of his fortune was the Milton Hershey School. As a result of his largesse, the school is today one of the wealthiest schools in the world, and the largest residential education program in the U.S.

But the years since Milton Hershey died have not been kind to his vision. The chocolate business, including the Hershey Company, has shifted from family-run enterprises to vast multi-national corporations and conglomerates. As the industry has consolidated into large monopolies and cartels, it has become fiercely competitive. The bottom line has become so dominant that the conditions on cocoa farms are almost Montezuma-like in their brutality. Only now it is the lives of children that are sacrificed to "guarantee" a good cocoa harvest.

The Chocolate Manufacturers Association, too, has changed. Now known as the Chocolate Council of the National Confectioners Association, its website (*www.thestoryofchocolate.com*) presents photos of smiling African workers and prominently announces, "Your chocolate has a past":

> The treat that now lies quietly in its wrapper carries a story of exotic places, long journeys and small families that raise delicate tropical fruit trees. As you peel back the wrapper, you're uncovering the cacao tree's seed—and joining people the world over who have turned to this mysterious food for ritual, medicine and sheer pleasure for the past 4,000 years.

No mention is ever made of child slavery, nor is any hint given that anything unsavory might be involved at any level of the chocolate business.

NO SWEETNESS HERE

For the large chocolate companies, the practice of buying cocoa from farms that employ abusive child-labor practices enables them to keep costs down and profits up. In 2010, the Hershey Company reported a 54 percent jump in profits because of what it called "improved supply-chain efficiencies." Such "efficiencies" allow Hershey's CEO David J. West to be paid an annual salary of $8 million, while buying cocoa from farms that work young people almost to death.

The reality of abusive labor conditions on West African cocoa farms is a longstanding problem for the entire chocolate industry. But while most of Hershey's primary competitors have at least taken steps to reduce or eliminate slavery and other forms of abusive child labor from their chocolate supply chains, Hershey has done almost nothing.

On September 13, 2010, on the occasion of founder Milton Hershey's 153rd birthday, the Hershey Company finally got around to issuing its first ever "Corporate Social Responsibility Report." Long on platitudes and promises, it was a classic example of the practice of "green-washing"—misleading the public into thinking a company's policies and products are socially responsible when, in fact, they are not.

Meanwhile, on that very same day, a coalition of public-interest nonprofit groups (Green America, Global Exchange, Oasis USA, and the International Labor Rights Forum) issued an in-depth counter-report, titled "Time to Raise the Bar: The Real Corporate Social Responsibility Report from the Hershey Company." This carefully researched report pointed out that the Hershey Company lags well behind its competitors in taking responsibility for the impact the company is having on the local communities from which it sources cocoa around the world.

Hershey is well aware that many smaller chocolate companies in the U.S. have for years purchased only Fair Trade Certified cocoa, thus ensuring that cocoa farmers earn enough to support their families, invest in their futures, and send their children to school. In 2006, Hershey bought the Dagoba Chocolate Company, an Oregon-based maker of organic chocolate whose entire line of drinking chocolate, syrup, and cacao powder is certified Fair Trade. But Hershey claims that, although this is possible for smaller companies, it would be impossible for a company as large as it is.

"Time to Raise the Bar" makes it crystal clear that it's not just the smaller companies that have taken meaningful steps. "Many of the largest global chocolate corporations," says the report, "are increasingly sourcing cocoa beans that have been certified by independent organizations to meet various labor, social, and environment standards. But there has been one major exception to this trend: the Hershey Company."

Other large companies publicly identify their sources of cocoa. But not Hershey. Other companies employ third-party certification for the cocoa they source from West Africa. But not Hershey.

Cadbury Dairy Milk in the U.K., for example, was the first major brand to make all of its chocolate Fair Trade Certified. The company not only converted its top-selling chocolate bar to Fair Trade, it also extended its Fair Trade Certified Dairy Milk Bar to Australia, Canada, Ireland, and New Zealand.

Ben & Jerry's has taken it a step further. The company has not only agreed to achieve Fair Trade certification for all its cocoa by 2013, but has also pledged Fair Trade certification for all of its other ingredients that are eligible for such certification. Even Kraft Foods and Mars, hardly icons of social responsibility, have begun to purchase cocoa certified by the Rainforest Alliance to be free from the use of forced labor, child labor, or discrimination.

If other companies can do it, why can't Hershey? Do they think it's okay that children are abducted and then sold as slaves to Ivory Coast cocoa farmers? Do you think it's okay? Here's what you can do:

- Purchase organic chocolate. At present, no organic cocoa beans are coming from Ivory Coast, so organic chocolate is unlikely to be tainted by slavery.

- Purchase chocolate products from companies that only use cocoa that has definitively not been produced with slave labor. These companies include Clif Bar, Cloud 9, Dagoba Organic Chocolate, Denman Island Chocolate, Divine Chocolate, Equal Exchange, Gardners Candies, Green & Black's, John & Kira's, Kailua Candy Company, Koppers

Chocolate, L.A. Burdick Chocolates, Montezuma's Chocolates, NewLeaf Chocolates, Newman's Own Organics, Omanhene Cocoa Bean Company, Rapunzel Pure Organics, Shaman Chocolates, Sweet Earth Chocolates, Taza Chocolate, Endangered Species Chocolate, and Theo Chocolate.

- Watch the video at *www.youtube.com/watch?v=CK5K-aHyxcE*.

- Sign a petition and tell Hershey to stop using child and forced labor. You can find the petition online at: *www.raisethebarhershey.org.*

- Call Hershey and tell them to stop using child and forced labor at (800) 468-1714; dial 0, then 3.

- Go to *www.chainstorereaction.com* to send an email to Hershey.

- Get a DVD copy of the film *The Dark Side of Chocolate*, along with information about Fair Trade, from the good people at Green America. Watch it, show it to your friends, and spread the word. *www.greenamerica.org/programs/fairtrade/MovieScreening.cfm*

- Tweet about this book and tell your friends to read it and take the Hershey online survey. The more people who do, the greater the chance Hershey will finally take responsibility for its actions and its impact.

14

Bitter Beans: Why Fair Trade Coffee Matters So Much

ALTHOUGH CHOCOLATE HAS GOTTEN the most publicity of late, it isn't the only American staple produced by slaves. Some coffee beans are also tainted by slavery. In addition to producing nearly half of the world's cocoa, Ivory Coast is the world's fourth-largest grower of Robusta coffee. Robusta beans are used for espresso and instant coffees. They are also blended with milder Arabica beans to make ground coffees.

Often, coffee and cocoa are grown together on the same farm. The tall cacao trees shade the shorter coffee bushes. On some Ivory Coast farms, child slaves harvest coffee beans as well as the cacao pods that yield cocoa beans. More than 7,000 tons of Ivory Coast coffee arrive in the U.S. each year.

Like cocoa beans, coffee beans picked by slaves are mixed with those picked by paid workers. Some coffee industry executives say the labor issue isn't their concern. "This industry isn't responsible for what happens in a foreign country," said Gary Goldstein of the National Coffee Association, which represents the companies that make Folgers, Maxwell House, Nescafé, and other brands.

The U.S. is the world's largest consumer of both chocolate and coffee. In fact, coffee is the second largest legal U.S. import—after oil. Fortunately, there is considerable momentum developing in this country and elsewhere behind the emergence of Fair Trade coffee.

According to the San Francisco–based Global Exchange:

> The best way to prevent child labor in the fields is to pay workers a living wage. . . . Most people in this country would rather buy a cup of coffee picked under fair trade conditions than sweatshop labor conditions. . . . Fair Trade Certified coffee is the first product being introduced in the United States with an independently monitored system to ensure that it was produced under fair labor conditions. . . . To become Fair Trade Certified, an importer must meet stringent international criteria [including] paying a minimum price per pound.

Paying a minimum price to growers is a major step, because coffee prices on the world market currently are so low that they trap many coffee farmers in an inescapable cycle of poverty, debt, and hunger. Ten years ago, the world coffee economy was worth $30 billion—of which producers received $12 billion, or 40 percent. But today, the world market has grown to be worth more than $50 billion—of which producers receive just $8 billion, or 16 percent. Although they have not lowered consumer prices, coffee companies are paying far less for the beans they use. This creates, at best, sweatshops in the field and, at worst, the conditions that breed human slavery.

Many of the people growing coffee work exceedingly long hours for less than $600 per year, while others are enslaved and paid nothing. Meanwhile, Irene Rosenfeld, CEO of Kraft Foods, the parent company of Maxwell House Coffee, is paid more than $26 million a year—which is a lot, but not as much as Howard D. Schultz, CEO of Starbucks, who receives more than $30 million a year. It's not easy for most consumers to stomach the contrast between the gruesome reality of slave labor and salaries that enable CEOs to live like emperors.

Fair Trade, whether it's coffee or chocolate, means an equitable partnership between consumers in North America and producers in Asia, Africa, Latin America, and the Caribbean. It means that farmers' cooperatives around the world can count on a stable and reliable living wage. When consumers purchase Fair Trade coffee or chocolate, they know that their money is going to local farmers who can then invest it in healthcare, education, environmental stewardship, community development, and economic independence. They know that they are not financing a system in which destitute farmers are struggling to survive and even resorting to child slavery.

Kevin Bales, director of Free the Slaves, reminds us that:

> [Consumers] can make a significant impact on world slavery just by stopping for a moment and asking themselves how that particular item got to be so cheap. The low cost of many items defies belief. Part of the reason things are so cheap is that the big chain stores buy huge quantities at huge discounts, and have designed their distribution systems to reduce overhead all along the product chain. But these economies of scale don't account for all of the cheapness. The bottom line is: oftentimes things are cheap because slaves helped produce them.

Most Western consumers would avoid buying slave-produced goods, despite their lower price, if they could identify them. Like most consumers, I look for bargains, and don't always stop to ask why a product is so cheap. It is sobering to realize that by always looking for the best deal, I may be choosing slave-made products without knowing what I am buying.

We have reason for hope, however, based on how well most consumers respond to the challenge of slavery—when they know about it. Once people understand that slavery still exists, they are nearly unanimous in their desire to see it stopped. They are more than willing; they are eager to make choices that respect basic human rights and uphold the dignity of those whose toil brings us goods that enrich our lives.

Buying Fair Trade is a step we can all take toward a better world.

15

Pink KFC Buckets?

WE LIVE IN A WORLD of profound contradictions. Some things are just unbelievably strange. At times, I feel as if I've found a way to adapt to the weirdness of the world, and then along comes something that just boggles my mind.

The largest grassroots breast cancer advocacy group in the world, a group called Susan G. Komen for the Cure, partnered with the fast-food chain KFC in a national Buckets for the Cure campaign in 2010.

KFC is taking every chance it can manufacture to trumpet its donation of fifty cents to Komen for every pink bucket of chicken sold.

For its part, Komen announced on its website that "KFC and Susan G. Komen for the Cure are teaming up . . . to . . . spread educational messaging via a major national campaign which will reach thousands of communities served by nearly 5,000 KFC restaurants."

Educational messaging indeed. How often do you think this "messaging" provides information about the critical importance a good diet plays in maintaining a healthy weight and preventing cancer? How often do you think it refers in any way to the many studies that, according to the National Cancer Institute's website, "have shown that an increased risk of developing colorectal, pancreatic, and breast cancer is associated with high intakes of well-done, fried, or barbecued meats"?

If you guessed zero, you're right.

Meanwhile, the American Institute for Cancer Research reports that 60 to 70 percent of all cancers can be prevented with lifestyle changes. Their number one dietary recommendation is: "Choose predominantly plant-based diets rich in a variety of vegetables and fruits, legumes and minimally processed starchy staple foods." Does that sound like pink buckets of fried chicken?

Pardon me for being cynical, but I have to ask: If Komen is going to partner with KFC, why not take it a step further and partner with a cigarette company? They could sell pink packages of cigarettes, donating a few cents from each pack while claiming, "Each pack you smoke brings us closer to the day cancer is vanquished forever."

Whose brilliant idea was it that buying fried chicken by the bucket is an effective way to fight breast cancer? One breast cancer advocacy group, Breast Cancer Action, thought the Komen/KFC campaign to be so egregious that they called it "pink-washing," another sad example of commercialism draped in pink ribbons. "Make no mistake," they said, "every pink bucket purchase will do more to benefit KFC's bottom line than it will to cure breast cancer."

Of course, it's not hard to understand KFC's motives. They want to make money and look good. But recent publicity the company has been getting hasn't been helping. For one thing, the company keeps taking hits for the unhealthiness of its food. Just weeks before launching its Pink Buckets campaign, KFC came out with its new Double Down sandwiches. The products were derided by just about every public health organization for their staggering levels of salt, calories, and artery-clogging fat.

Then there's the squeamish matter of the treatment of the birds that end up in KFC's buckets, pink or otherwise. People for the Ethical Treatment of Animals (PETA) has an entire website devoted to what they call Kentucky Fried Cruelty, but you don't have to be an animal activist to be horrified by how the company treats chickens, once you lift the veil of the company's PR and see what actually takes place.

When PETA sent investigators with hidden cameras into a KFC "Supplier of the Year" slaughterhouse in Moorefield, West Virginia, what they found was enough to make KFC choke on its own pink publicity stunts. Workers were caught on video stomping on chickens, kicking them, and violently slamming them against floors and walls. Workers were also filmed ripping the animals' beaks off, twisting their heads off, spitting tobacco into their eyes and mouths, spray-painting their faces, and squeezing their bodies so hard that the birds expelled feces—all while the chickens were still alive.

Dan Rather echoed the views of many who saw the footage when he said on the *CBS Evening News,* "There's no mistaking what the video depicts: cruelty to animals, chickens horribly mistreated before they're slaughtered for a fast-food chain."

KFC, naturally, did everything they could to keep the footage from being aired, but their efforts failed. In fact, the video from the investigation ended up being broadcast by TV stations around the world, as well as on all three national evening news shows, *Good Morning America,* and every one of the major cable news networks. In addition, more than a million people subsequently watched the footage on PETA's website.

It wasn't just animal activists who condemned the fast-food chain for the level of animal cruelty displayed at KFC's "Supplier of the Year" slaughterhouse. Dr. Temple Grandin, perhaps the meat industry's leading farmed-animal welfare expert, said: "The behavior of the plant employees was atrocious." Dr. Ian Duncan, Professor of Applied Ethology at the University of Guelph and an original member of KFC's own animal welfare advisory council, wrote: "This tape depicts scenes of the worst cruelty I have ever witnessed against chickens . . . and it is extremely hard to accept that this is occurring in the United States of America."

KFC claims, on its website, that its animal welfare advisory council "has been a key factor in formulating our animal welfare program." But Dr. Duncan, along with five other former members of KFC's animal welfare advisory council, says otherwise. They all resigned in disgust over the company's refusal to take animal welfare seriously. Adele Douglass, one of those who resigned, said in an SEC filing reported on by the *Chicago Tribune* that KFC "never had any meetings. They never asked any advice, and then they touted to the press that they had this animal welfare advisory committee. I felt like I was being used."

You can see why KFC would be eager to jump on any chance to improve its public image, and why the company would want to capitalize on any opportunity to associate itself in the public mind with the fight against breast cancer. What's far more mystifying is why an organization with as much public trust as Susan B. Komen for the Cure would jeopardize public confidence in its authenticity. As someone once said, it takes a lifetime to build a reputation, but only fifteen minutes to lose it.

One thing is hard to dispute. In partnering with KFC, Susan B. Komen for the Cure has shown itself to be numbingly oblivious to the role of diet in cancer prevention.

If you want to support an organization fighting breast cancer, you may want to know about the little-known but extraordinary Pine Street Foundation. While everyone wants to detect breast cancer as early as possible, the Pine Street Foundation has been developing a remarkable alternative to mammograms. Susan B. Komen for the Cure, you may know, has been one of the foremost proponents of mammograms, suggesting their use for women as young as twenty-five. But mammograms involve subjecting a woman's breast to radiation; thus, if repeated too often, they can actually raise the risk of breast cancer.

In a large international collaboration, the Pine Street Foundation has been studying the ability of dogs to use their remarkable sense of smell for the early detection of lung and breast cancer. The work is based on the fact that cancer cells emit different metabolic waste products than normal cells, and the differences between these can be detected by a dog's keen sense of smell, even in the early stages of the disease. So far, the dogs' ability to identify or rule out lung and breast cancer correctly, at both early and late stages, has been around 90 percent—approximately the same accuracy rate as mammograms, with none of the radiation. In one study involving more than 12,000 separate scent trials, for example, dogs were able to identify lung and breast cancer patients by smelling samples of their breath. The dogs' performance was not affected by the disease stage of cancer patients, nor by their age, or by smoking or recently eaten food.

I've met the dogs involved in these studies (Portuguese water dogs, and yellow and black Labrador retrievers) and I know the people who have designed and undertaken these studies, and I am honestly quite impressed. Unfortunately, it is not yet possible to be "screened" by the dogs to see if you have cancer, but there is every hope that the concepts explored in this research will lead in the future to cancer-screening methods that are more accurate than mammograms, and less harmful.

The work of the Pine Street Foundation is a good example of the many new and hopeful possibilities that are emerging. Every day, there are more people and more groups blazing a path to healthy food, real prevention, and less toxic yet more effective approaches to treatment. The Cancer Project, for example, promotes cancer prevention, in particular by advocating for nutritional approaches that reduce cancer risk. Breast Cancer Action carries the voices of people affected by breast cancer out to inspire and compel the changes necessary to end the breast cancer epidemic. And Beyond Pesticides works to protect public health and the environment while leading the transition to a more safe and sustainable world.

Vibrant, grounded, and inspiring, these groups and many others like them are pointing in a healthy and sane direction. In a time when KFC has become the poster company for pink-washing, they stand before us as true examples of the way to health, sanity, and human fulfillment.

16

Super Size Me

Morgan Spurlock sought to find out just how bad McDonald's food is in his 2004 documentary *Super Size Me*. In his film, I was interviewed and spoke about the role McDonald's food is playing in our epidemic of obesity and diabetes.

For thirty days, Spurlock ate only McDonald's food. All of us involved in the film, including Spurlock's doctors, were shocked at the amount that his health deteriorated in such a short time. Before the thirty days started, we each predicted what changes we expected to see in his weight, cholesterol levels, liver enzymes, and other biomarkers, but every one of us substantially underestimated how severely his health would be jeopardized. It turned out that in thirty days, the then thirty-two-year-old man gained twenty-five pounds, his cholesterol levels rose dangerously as did fatty accumulations in his liver, and he experienced mood swings, depression, heart palpitations, and sexual dysfunction.

Some have said Spurlock was an idiot for eating that way, and it's true that he did himself some major damage in those thirty days. But I've always felt the suffering he took upon himself by eating all his meals for that month at McDonald's was admirable, because it served to warn millions of the all-too-real health dangers of eating too much fast food.

Super Size Me struck a chord with a lot of people, as it became one of the highest-grossing documentaries of all time and was nominated for an Academy Award for Best Documentary Feature. And more important, it changed the eating habits of countless people.

In 2010, a group of physicians and other health professionals produced a short (thirty-nine-second) ad that may have been one of the more controversial in advertising history. The Washington, DC–based group Physicians Committee for Responsible Medicine (PCRM)'s "Consequences" ad took dead aim at McDonald's high-fat menu. The provocative ad quickly became a story unto itself, because in only a few days it generated nearly one million views on YouTube, and was covered by newspapers and broadcast media around the world, including *The Wall Street Journal*, U.K.'s *The Guardian*, CNN, *The New York Times*, and hundreds of other media outlets. You can see it on YouTube by searching for "PCRM Consequences."

The ad ends by telling us to "make it vegetarian," making it obvious that PCRM has a pro-vegetarian orientation. But with good reason. The evidence is consistent and compelling that vegetarians suffer less from the diseases associated with the typical Western diet. Vegetarians have repeatedly been shown to have lower rates of obesity, coronary heart disease, hypertension, type-2 diabetes, diverticular disease, constipation, and gallstones. They also have lower rates of many kinds of cancer, including colon cancer and hormone-dependent cancers like prostate, breast, uterine, and ovarian cancer.

Do you have to be a strict vegetarian to enjoy the considerable health benefits of a vegetarian diet? No, you do not. What's important is to eat a plant-strong diet, with a high percentage of your calories coming from whole foods like fruits, vegetables, and whole grains, and a low percentage coming from processed foods, sugars, unhealthy fats, and animal products.

The standard American diet—in which 62 percent of calories come from processed foods, 25 percent from animal products, and only 5 percent from fruits and vegetables—is nothing less than a health travesty. Our fast-food culture has produced a population with widespread chronic illness and is a primary reason that healthcare costs are taking a devastating toll on just about everyone.

The annual health insurance premiums paid by the average American family now exceed the gross annual income of a full-time minimum-wage worker. Every thirty seconds, someone in the U.S. files for bankruptcy due to the costs of treating a health problem.

Medical care costs in the U.S. have not always been this excessive. In 2011, we spent more than $2.5 trillion on medical care. But in 1950, five years before Ray Kroc opened the first franchised McDonald's restaurant, Americans only spent $8.4 billion ($70 billion in today's dollars). The population has increased since then, but even after adjusting for inflation, we now spend as much on healthcare every ten days as we did in the entire year of 1950.

Has this enormous increase in spending made us healthier? Earlier this year, when the World Health Organization assessed the overall health outcomes of different nations, it placed thirty-six other nations ahead of the United States.

Today, we have an epidemic of largely preventable diseases. To these illnesses, Americans are losing not only their health but also their life savings. Meanwhile, the evidence keeps growing that the path to improved health lies in eating more vegetables, fruits, whole grains, and legumes, and eating far less processed foods, sugars, and animal products.

It's striking to me that, in all the heated debates we have had about healthcare reform, one basic fact has rarely been discussed—the one thing that could dramatically bring down the costs of healthcare while improving the health of our people. Studies have shown that 50 to 70 percent of the nation's healthcare costs are preventable, and the single most effective step most people can take to improve their health is to eat a healthier diet. If Americans stopped overeating, stopped eating unhealthy foods, and instead ate more foods with higher nutrient densities and cancer-protective properties, we could have a more affordable, sustainable, and effective healthcare system.

Is it McDonald's fault that more than 63 percent of Americans are overweight or obese, making us the fattest nation in the history of the world? I don't think so, because each of us is responsible for what we put in our mouths and in the mouths of our children. And many other fast-food chains serve food that is just as harmful.

But McDonald's plays a significant role in generating our national appetite for unhealthy foods. McDonald's is by far the largest food advertiser in the country, spending more than one billion dollars a year on direct media advertising.

Much of McDonald's advertising is aimed at children, and it's been effective. Every month, approximately nine out of ten American children eat at a McDonald's restaurant. Most U.S. children can recognize McDonald's before they can speak. Tragically, one in every three children born this year in the U.S. will develop diabetes in their lifetime.

Of course, fast food is not the only cause of the tragic rise in obesity and diabetes in our society. Our culture has become pathologically sedentary. Watching television and sitting in front of computer monitors for hour upon hour doesn't help. But the high-sugar and high-fat foods sold by McDonald's and other fast-food restaurants are certainly a major part of the problem. You would have to walk for seven hours without stopping to burn off the calories from a Big Mac, a Coke, and an order of fries.

17

The Battle for Our Children

WE WORRY SO MUCH about the many dangers to our children—about drugs and pedophiles and violence. But we often take for granted what may very well be the greatest danger of all to their health—the hundreds of billions of dollars spent each year on ads designed to get them hooked on junk food.

That's why I think it's newsworthy that, in 2011, more than 550 health professionals and organizations signed an open letter to McDonald's imploring the fast-food giant to stop marketing junk food to children. Many major metropolitan newspapers across the country ran full-page notices featuring the letter.

The letter didn't ask McDonald's to stop *selling* junk food to children. It only asked them to stop *aggressively advertising* these foods to children.

The letter campaign, organized by the nonprofit watchdog group Corporate Accountability International, did not meet with universal applause. Critics tried to dismiss it as just another attempt to limit consumer freedom, just another effort by the food police to dictate what you and your children can eat.

McDonald's food may be junk, they said, but it's a personal choice. No one is physically forcing children to eat Big Macs. Where are parents anyway? Why don't they exert their authority and take responsibility? Are they just looking for someone other than themselves to blame because their children are fat and unhealthy?

Of course, no one—not even McDonald's—doubts that we are witnessing an escalating epidemic of obesity and diet-related disease in children. Some try to blame a lack of exercise, but many studies show that exercise levels in children haven't changed much in the past two decades. What, then, lies at the root of the crisis?

The critics of the ad campaign, and McDonald's itself, place the blame for the situation squarely on the shoulders of parents. The problem, they say, is a breakdown in parental responsibility.

Like the critics, I am a staunch advocate of parental responsibility. But I part company with them here and whole-heartedly endorse the effort to ban junk-food advertising to children because McDonald's and other junk-food ads are deliberately designed to compromise parental authority. The advertising industry calls it "the pester factor." The PR companies who produce these ads speak casually of making children "obnoxious," of getting them to "drive their parents crazy."

The goal is to get children to want junk food so much that they nag their parents to take them to McDonald's and to buy them other foods they have seen advertised, eventually breaking down parents' resistance. In the face of the relentless barrage of these advertisements, how many parents are able to hold their ground?

The "pester factor" has enormous economic implications. Advertisers estimate that one out of three fast-food trips take place as a result of a child's nagging.

The marketing strategy is clever and effective, but it's insidious. Traditionally, it has been parents who have had the responsibility for decisions about what their children eat. But McDonald's and other fast-food companies spend billions of dollars a year on ad campaigns that target children, with the goal of taking that responsibility away from the parents and shifting it onto the children themselves. In this way, the ads not only promote the consumption of junk food, with all the baneful health consequences we are witnessing today. What may be even worse is that, at the same time, this kind of marketing systematically undermines the role of the parents in selecting healthy foods for their children. The continual onslaught of such ads erodes the respect parents have for themselves and the respect they command from their children.

What makes junk-food ads targeting children even more damaging is that young children are not capable of understanding that the advertising is intended to manipulate their feelings and alter their behavior. Given that children can't comprehend the persuasive intent behind ads, is it exploitive to advertise unhealthy foods to them? Should it even be legal?

Calling on McDonald's CEO and President Jim Skinner to "stop marketing junk food to kids," the letter was signed by a veritable Who's Who of luminaries in the world of healthy eating and disease prevention, including authors Andrew Weil and T. Colin Campbell. Other signatories include David L. Katz, Director of the Yale Prevention Research Center and editor-in-chief of *Child Obesity*; Robert S. Lawrence, Director of the Center for a Livable Future, Johns Hopkins Bloomberg School of Public Health; Marion Nestle, Paulette Goodard Professor in the Department of Nutrition, Food Studies and Public Health, and Professor of Sociology at New York University; and Walter Willett, Chairman of the Department of Nutrition, Harvard School of Public Health. The letter states:

> As health professionals engaged directly in the largest preventable health crisis facing this country, we ask that you stop marketing junk food to children.
>
> The rates of sick children are staggering. Ballooning health care costs and an overburdened health care system

make treatment more difficult than ever. And we know that reducing junk food marketing can significantly improve the health of kids.

Our community is devoted to caring for sick children and preventing illness through public education. But our efforts cannot compete with the hundreds of millions of dollars you spend each year directly marketing to kids.

Today, our private practices, pediatric clinics, and emergency rooms are filled with children suffering from conditions related to the food they eat. In the decades to come, one in three children will develop type-2 diabetes as a result of diets high in McDonald's-style junk food, according to the Centers for Disease Control and Prevention. This generation may be the first in U.S. history to live shorter lives than their parents.

The rise of health conditions like diabetes and heart disease mirrors the growth of your business—growth driven in large part by children's marketing . . .

While acknowledging that fast food is unhealthy, you pin responsibility for the epidemic of diet related disease on a breakdown in parental responsibility . . .

Even when parents resist the "nag effect" cultivated by McDonald's to access the $40–50 billion in annual purchases that children under 12 control, advertising creates brand loyalties that persist into adulthood . . .

We ask that you . . . retire your marketing promotions for food high in salt, fat, sugar, and calories to children . . .

McDonald's claims it's doing enough already by being part of the Children's Food and Beverage Advertising Initiative. But this program is merely an entirely voluntary statement, produced by representatives from Burger King, Coca-Cola,

Hershey, Mars, Nestlé, and PepsiCo, along with McDonald's. As you can imagine, the "pledges" made by various companies under the Initiative have done absolutely nothing to stem the tide of marketing junk food to children.

And why would McDonald's want to cease this practice voluntarily? In 2009, McDonald's CEO and President Jim Skinner took home more than $17 million in compensation for his time and efforts.

Meanwhile his company spends millions of dollars every single day on ads geared to children.

If we love our children, why do we let corporations pummel them with sophisticated ads that make them crave foods that will damage their health?

These ads are designed to get children hooked. And they are designed to undermine parental authority. The harm is serious, and it's life-long.

Isn't it time that we protect our families and ban this kind of advertising?

18

The Vitaminwater Deception

When this article first appeared on HuffingtonPost *in 2010, it was read by nearly a million people, and quickly became the most widely viewed serious news post in the history of the site. Coca-Cola was not pleased.*

Now here's something you wouldn't expect. Coca-Cola is being sued by a non-profit public interest group on the grounds that the company's vitaminwater products make unwarranted health claims. No surprise there. But how do you think the company is defending itself?

In a staggering feat of twisted logic, lawyers for Coca-Cola are defending the lawsuit by asserting that "no consumer could reasonably be misled into thinking vitaminwater was a healthy beverage."

Does this mean that you'd have to be an unreasonable person to think that a product named vitaminwater, a product that has been heavily and aggressively marketed as a healthy beverage, actually had health benefits?

Or does it mean that it's okay for a corporation to lie about its products, as long as they can then turn around and claim that no one actually believes their lies?

In fact, the product is basically sugar-water, to which about a penny's worth of synthetic vitamins have been added.

And the amount of sugar is not trivial. A bottle of vitamin-water contains 33 grams of sugar, making it more akin to a soft drink than to a healthy beverage.

Is any harm being done by this marketing ploy? After all, some might say consumers are at least getting some vitamins, and there isn't as much sugar in vitaminwater as there is in regular Coke.

True. But about 35 percent of Americans are now considered medically obese. Two-thirds of Americans are overweight. Health experts tend to disagree about almost everything, but they all concur that added sugars play a key role in the obesity epidemic, a problem that now leads to more medical costs than smoking.

How many people with weight problems have consumed products like vitaminwater in the mistaken belief that the product provides nutritional benefits and carries no caloric consequences? How many have thought that consuming vitaminwater is a smart choice from a weight-loss perspective? The very name vitaminwater suggests that the product is simply water with added nutrients, disguising the fact that it's actually full of added sugar.

The truth is that, when it comes to weight loss, what you drink may be even more important than what you eat. Americans now get nearly 25 percent of their calories from liquids. In 2009, researchers at the Johns Hopkins Bloomberg School of Public Health published a report in *The American Journal of Clinical Nutrition* that found that the quickest and most reliable way to lose weight is to cut down on liquid calorie consumption. And the best way to do that is to reduce or eliminate beverages that contain added sugar.

Meanwhile, Coca-Cola has invested billions of dollars in its vitaminwater line, paying basketball stars like Kobe Bryant and Lebron James to appear in ads that emphatically state that these products are a healthy way for consumers to hydrate. When Lebron James held his much ballyhooed TV special to announce his decision to join the Miami Heat, many corporations paid millions in an attempt to capitalize on the event. But it was vitaminwater that had the most prominent role throughout the show.

The lawsuit, brought by the Center for Science in the Public Interest, alleges that vitaminwater labels and advertising are filled with "deceptive and unsubstantiated claims." In his recent fifty-five-page ruling, Federal Judge John Gleeson (U.S. District Court for the Eastern District of New York), wrote: "At oral arguments, defendants (Coca-Cola) suggested that no consumer could reasonably be misled into thinking vitaminwater was a healthy beverage." Noting that the soft drink giant wasn't claiming the lawsuit was wrong on factual grounds, the judge wrote: "Accordingly, I must accept the factual allegations in the complaint as true."

I still can't get over the bizarre audacity of Coke's legal case. Forced to defend themselves in court, they acknowledged that vitaminwater isn't a healthy product. But they argued that advertising it as a health beverage isn't false advertising, because no one could possibly believe such a ridiculous claim.

I guess that's why they spend hundreds of millions of dollars advertising the product, saying it will keep you "healthy as a horse," and will bring about a "healthy state of physical and mental well-being."

Why do we allow companies like Coca-Cola to tell us that drinking a bottle of sugar water with a few added water-soluble vitamins is a legitimate way to meet our nutritional needs?

Here's what I suggest: If you're looking for a healthy and far less expensive way to hydrate, try drinking water. If you want to flavor the water you drink, try adding the juice of a lemon and a small amount of honey or maple syrup to a quart of water. Another alternative is to mix one part lemonade or fruit juice to three or four parts water. Or drink green tea, hot or chilled, adding lemon and a small amount of sweetener if you like. If you want to jazz it up, try one-half fruit juice, one-half carbonated water.

If your tap water tastes bad or you suspect it may contain lead or other contaminants, get a water filter that fits under the sink or attaches to the tap.

And it's probably not the best idea to rely on a soft drink company for your vitamins and other essential nutrients. A plant-strong diet with lots of vegetables and fruits will provide you with what you need far more reliably, far more consistently—and far more honestly.

PART FOUR

Being Human in This Troubled World

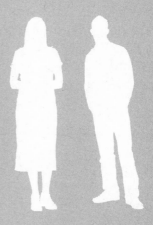

19

Remembering How Much
Relationships Matter

I BELIEVE THAT, VERY OFTEN, there is a strong connection between the quality of the food a person eats and the quality of the life they are able to live. As a result, I try to be discerning about what I eat. For the most part, I consume only healthy, natural foods. I eat more fresh vegetables, and particularly more greens, than just about anyone else I know. I even have a T-shirt that says "Plant Strong" on one side, and "Eat Greens" on the other.

I am sure it won't surprise you to learn that I have friends and relatives, on the other hand, who are less conscientious in their choices.

Or at least that's how I see it—that they are less conscientious—although they would probably say it differently. In fact, they might say that they are less obsessive about their food choices, or that they are more relaxed and easy-going about it all.

Regardless of how you look at it, however, we definitely have our differences. And I've been thinking, lately, about how I respond to these differences. It's not always easy.

I try to be in touch with my respect for other people's right to make their own choices. No one likes to feel defensive or criticized. I want to remember that each of us chooses our own path in life. At the same time, I care about these people and want them to know all the joys of a long and healthy life. There is an art to expressing caring in a way that gives the optimal opportunity for people to feel supported, not judged.

There is a young man in the town where I live who may not have fully mastered this art. He often seems to make it his business to lecture other people about what's wrong with their lifestyle choices.

One day, I found myself standing behind him at the checkout stand of the local health food store. A mother with three small children, obviously looking stressed, was in line in front of him. The young man did not know the woman, but that did not stop him. He began pointing disapprovingly at the items she was buying, as they sat on the conveyor belt approaching the cash register.

"Are you aware," he scolded her loudly, "how much damage you are doing to your children by feeding them junk food?" I looked at the foods and, frankly, they didn't look all that bad to me. I saw bananas, apples, canned beans, chocolate milk, pasta sauce, a couple bags of corn chips, and a few other items.

He glared at a package of organic cookies, and none-too-kindly asked: "Do you know how much sugar is in those cookies? Don't you realize how bad that is?"

Seeing him act this way, I was poignantly reminded of something Martin Luther King once said: "You have no moral authority with those who can feel your underlying contempt."

I thought there was no way the mother would listen to him, considering how disdainfully he spoke to her. But then it occurred to me, and I must say that it was a humbling experience, that I was filled with just as much underlying contempt as he was—only mine was directed at him.

There is a saying that we always accuse others of our own vices. We project our shadow onto others, and then find fault with them for it. What we judge in others is often what we have disowned in ourselves.

Was it possible that this man, in his arrogance, was a mirror of something I didn't like in myself?

I can, at times, be so zealous in my beliefs that I become rigid and uncaring toward others. I've seen myself become so narrow-minded and identified with my own opinions that I can't hear others, can't see any validity in viewpoints that don't reinforce my own. I've seen myself be harshly judgmental of others without even thinking about what it would be like to walk a mile in their moccasins. I've seen myself be self-righteous even when doing so is clearly undermining my relationships.

It was not pleasant to see my own shortcomings mirrored in someone whose actions I didn't like, but it served a purpose. It put me back in touch with what I need to work on in myself. It released me, at least a little bit, from my contempt for him, and brought me into contact with some of the central questions that I live with on a daily basis.

How can I be true to myself and also as unconditionally loving toward others as possible? How can I stay centered on my path, while also honoring others when they have different paths? How can I live passionately according to my values and principles, while also being respectful of others who make other kinds of choices?

I wasn't sure if I wanted to interact with the young man, but as I thought of doing so, the golden rule came to mind: Do unto others as you would like them to do unto you. Okay then, how would I like someone to relate to me when I am mired in pompous self-importance? Was it possible for me to relate to him and to what he was doing genuinely and with compassion rather than contempt?

The harried mother wheeled her shopping cart out the door and made her way toward the parking lot, children in tow. The cashier began ringing up the groceries of the young man in front of me.

"It seems as if you are quite health conscious," I reflected.

"That's for sure," he said proudly. "I eat only raw, organic, locally grown food." He gestured toward the food he was purchasing, obviously pleased with himself.

"How's it working for you?" I asked.

"Fantastic!" he declared, as though he were the winner in some kind of competition.

"I'm glad to hear it," I said softly. He cracked a smile and, for the first time, looked at me. I sensed I might have an opening, so I decided to take a risk

"I noticed what you said to the lady with the kids."

"Yes, well, somebody had to straighten her out."

"She seemed embarrassed by what you said."

"She should be."

"Do you want to know what I noticed?" I asked.

"I guess so," he said. He seemed uncertain, but I decided to take this as an invitation.

"I know you wanted to help her," I said. "At the same time, what I've learned from plenty of my own mistakes and my own experience is that shaming people is usually not the best way to encourage them. I find that what I appreciate tends to grow. That's why I like to acknowledge people for the positive choices they make. I've seen a lot of people feed their kids a lot worse things than what she was buying."

He seemed to be listening, but I wasn't sure.

"Maybe she deserves some credit and acknowledgment," I continued. "Who knows? Maybe she used to feed them Cocoa Puffs or fried bacon for breakfast, like many mothers in this country do, and now she's making an effort to do better. Maybe she needs to be appreciated for the healthy choices she's making more than she needs to be put down for not living up to someone else's standards."

I was concerned that my words might make him defensive, but he seemed pensive, calmer, and less full of himself. On the other hand, maybe he was just quiet because he was searching for a way to rebut what I had said. I wasn't sure how my little intervention had landed.

At that moment, the bagger placed the man's groceries in his cart and thanked him for shopping there. As the young man began to leave, he turned and glanced quickly at the items I was purchasing, which were now displayed on the counter. Along with plenty of fresh vegetables and fresh fruit, there was also a bag of organic potato chips, which I was tempted to snatch and hide. More important—and this is what obviously caught his eye—there were several bars of my favorite dark chocolate.

For a moment, I thought I was going to get the same treatment he had given the mother, but then I saw the expression on his face change to something like relief. "I like that type of chocolate, too," he said, and there was actual friendliness in his voice. "It's organic and Fair Trade."

"Yes," I said, "it is. And delicious."

"Yes, delicious," he said, smiling widely. "Have a great day."

"You too."

I was glad that I hadn't obeyed my first impulse, which had been to reprimand him for the way he had spoken to the hassled mother. I was glad I had found a way to talk with him, rather than at him.

When we react with judgment, when we seek to punish and shame those who don't live up to our ideals, we only perpetuate cycles of suffering.

20

Do Friends Let Friends
Eat Junk Food?

I HAVE WRITTEN EIGHT BOOKS advocating a healthier way of
life and a more nutritious diet. These books have sold millions of copies, and have been translated into about thirty
languages, so I know that my work has touched many lives.
My first book, *Diet for a New America*, was originally published in 1987, before the advent of email and the Internet.
I received more than 60,000 letters (yes, actual letters) from
readers thanking me for the inspiration and support they felt
they had gotten from the book. To do this work has been
a privilege, and I am grateful for the opportunities I have
had to help people take responsibility for their health and for
their relationship with the wider Earth community.

Nonetheless, like most people, I have friends and family
members who aren't much interested in what I have to say.
And, of course, I am surrounded—as we all are—by a culture
of processed and industrialized food, sold to us by corporations that bombard us from our earliest childhood with ads
pushing us to consume food-like substances that are egre-
giously high in sugar, bad fats, additives, and calories virtually devoid of nutrition.

I'm often asked how I relate to people who apparently
aren't interested in taking any responsibility for healthy food

choices. Usually, I don't try too hard with such people. My books are available, as are many other fine books and documentaries supporting people in eating a diet that is higher in nutrition. But of course, if they are family members or friends, it's not so easy to simply walk away. And sometimes, it's a real struggle.

I try to accept these struggles with as much grace as possible, and to remember that, even if I dislike someone's actions, I can still retain a connection to their hearts.

One of my friends suffers from chronic depression. He eats a diet that consists primarily of French fries, soft drinks, and burgers. I'm not sure he would recognize a vegetable if he saw one. Because he knows that I eat much more healthfully, he feels a need from time to time to justify his eating habits to me. The last time that happened, he repeated something that I've often heard him say:

"Things are so bad, I may as well try and get a little pleasure."

"Yes," I replied on this particular occasion, knowing of his suffering and wanting to be kind, but also knowing that I needed to say something that didn't collude with his self-pity. "I've heard you say that often. And I agree that is one way to look at it. Might you be open to hearing another possibility?"

He shrugged his shoulders. "Like what?"

"I hear you saying that life can be difficult, so why not take the little pleasures that are available."

"Yes, exactly," he replied.

"Well, on the other hand, do you think it might be possible for you to get a *lot* of pleasure out of life by taking better care of yourself and being more healthy and vibrant?"

He did not seem hopeful. For today, anyway, his cynicism prevailed. I gave him a hug and told him that whatever he did, I would still love him. I didn't feel that my words had been useful to him, but I did feel my caring for him and also that I was being true to myself, so I was glad that I had spoken up.

When we parted that day, I offered him a simple prayer: May you live from your deepest truth in a way that enables you to thrive.

I have another friend who is more than 100 pounds over-weight, and who frequently complains about how bad she feels and how little energy she has. She starts her day with donuts and coffee for breakfast, and refers to her kitchen as "Junk Food Central." One day, I watched her eat the entire contents of an extra-large bag of Oreo cookies. She then recited her mantra, the thing she says repeatedly to justify her unhealthy eating patterns:

"Why deprive myself?" she says. "You only live once."

Usually, when she says that, I just smile and wish her a good day. I know that her life is difficult, and I know also that she is so set in her ways that there really isn't much point in saying anything. But on this particular day, watching her gorge herself on Oreos was too much for me. I couldn't stay silent any longer.

"If you only live once," I said, "wouldn't it make more sense to eat healthier food so you could get the most out of this one life by feeling more alive and having more energy?"

As you can see, I can be a bit of a pest. It's a wonder my friends stick around. In this case, my words did not fall on receptive ears.

"Health," she retorted loudly, "is just a matter of karma and genetics. What you eat is at most 1 percent of it."

I was quiet for awhile. I didn't see much point in arguing with her. But she wouldn't let it rest.

"What do you say to that?" she demanded.

"I'm just thinking," I answered slowly, "about how easy it is to be in denial without knowing it."

"Are you implying that I'm in denial?" she said testily.

"I don't know," I answered. "What do you think? Do you think there's the teeniest tiniest bit of a chance that you might be just a little bit?"

She picked up her kitchen towel and swatted me with it teasingly.

"Oh, John," she said. "Whatever am I going to do with you? You're unrelenting. But you really do care about me, don't you?"

At that moment I was glad that I'm tall. When we hugged, my long arms reached all the way around her. Our eyes caught, there was a moment of shared understanding, and we laughed.

May we all have the courage to change the things we can, the serenity to accept the things we can't, and the wisdom to know the difference.

21

Mike

MY COMMITMENT TO FIND a way to be helpful without judging others for poor food choices was sorely tested when a friend of mine came down with colon cancer. Not that my relationship with Mike had ever been particularly easy. He could be, to be perfectly frank, a bit of a pain. When we went out to eat, he always—knowing full well that I was a vegetarian and had written books on the subject—asked me whether I felt more like a steak or a hamburger. He always made a point of telling me during the meal how fabulous his meat or ice cream tasted, and made a display of offering to share it with me, all the while acting as if his doing so were motivated entirely by affection and generous concern for my well-being.

It wasn't only at restaurants that this kind of thing went on. Mike and I were running partners. When he outpaced me in the long-distance runs we sometimes took together, he announced triumphantly that his prowess was entirely due to the bacon he had eaten that morning. He did this, I am sure, even on those days when his breakfast had been granola.

But I was not about to let him get my goat. I just smiled and inwardly vowed that next time I would win. Not that I ever did. He had been a champion cross-country runner in high school, and was naturally gifted. I, on the other hand— well, let's just say I tried hard.

Still, I worried about him. Perhaps because physical things had always come easily to Mike, he seemed to take his health for granted. Aside from our runs, he didn't exercise much and, as time passed, he gained quite a bit of weight. He became less and less interested in running and eventually stopped altogether.

I chided him that it was obvious that he was terrified of losing to me and that the reason he no longer wanted to go for runs was that he simply wanted to avoid the inevitable experience of watching me cross the finish line ahead of him. His reply wasn't particularly subtle: "My ass, Mr. Bean-sprouts-for-breakfast. You couldn't beat me if I had to hop on one leg." Of course, he was wrong. I've never once eaten bean sprouts for breakfast.

Once I spoke to him about *ahimsa*, the practice of non-violence, the practice of living with compassion for all creatures.

"That sounds great," he answered. "I'm into ahimsa— ahimsa for myself. I'm not going to do violence to myself by denying myself a nice thick slice of roast beef. Want to join me?"

"No, thanks," I answered, softly. I didn't say any more. I didn't feel like arguing with him. I didn't want to create any more separation. I thought he was creating quite enough all by himself.

"No problem," he responded. "But don't forget that plants have consciousness, too." He pointed to my salad. "You're murdering those poor lettuce leaves."

On another occasion, I told him that I was concerned about his health. "I don't want to see you get sick." I mentioned that people who ate the way he did often developed chronic diseases like cancer.

"Maybe," he answered. "If it's in the cards, that's what's going to happen." He sounded resigned.

After Mike gained even more weight and stopped exercising entirely, his wife became concerned. "He's becoming increasingly irritable and short-tempered. What's worse, he doesn't talk to me anymore about what he's feeling, and spends all his free time on his computer."

We were seeing each other less and less, until one day Mike called and said he needed to talk to me. He had been to the doctor and had gotten some bad news. Could I come over?

Yes, I said, I'd be right over.

When I arrived, the atmosphere in their house was heavy and dark. His wife spoke first, and told me Mike had been diagnosed with a very serious form of colon cancer—Dukes' D. I knew what this meant. The cancer had already spread quite widely through the body.

The prognosis with Dukes' D is terrible. The five-year survival rate is about 5 percent, at best maybe 20 percent if liver metastases can be surgically removed.

They were scared. I listened, and my heart felt sick. Oh Mike, I thought, Oh Mike! Why didn't you listen? Didn't I tell you? Outwardly, I tried to listen and be supportive, but inside I was angry and hurt—angry at Mike for not taking better care of himself, angry at God for letting this happen, and angry at myself for not having been able to prevent it.

I listened as attentively as I could, and asked a few questions. They talked about his treatment options, and about the financial pressures they were dealing with. Not a word about diet. I stayed for dinner. Mike had a burger, fries, and a pint of ice cream. He seemed despondent.

For once, he didn't crack a single disparaging joke about my health-conscious ways, although for perhaps the first time I actually was wishing he would. I wanted him to be his old, stupid, teasing self. He may have been a jerk, but we were buddies, pals, compadres, friends. Oh, Mike.

I was hurting and I wanted to be in denial. I didn't want to face what was happening. I wanted the old Mike back, even if he was a jerk.

In the weeks that followed, Mike underwent surgery and then chemotherapy. He was having a terribly hard time with nausea, abdominal pain, vomiting, diarrhea, and a host of other kinds of distress, but he pinned his hopes for a cure on the drugs. He made it clear that he didn't want to discuss alternative or complementary treatments.

It was hard for me not to be critical. When Mike complained about how helpless he felt, I tried to be understanding and to help him make intelligent and grounded choices, but inside I was thinking: "Why didn't you think about that before? What do you expect when you eat the way you have?" He said he was at last cleaning up his diet, but I wasn't convinced. As far as I could tell, he was still eating the same junk he had always eaten.

Mike's last days weren't pleasant or comfortable. But there was one thing that happened that stands out for me, as I look back on it now. I don't want to make too much of this, but to me it feels important.

One of the last times I saw him, Mike said to me: "Thank you for not pushing your trip on me. I hate vegetables, that's all there is to it."

"I appreciate your saying that. But honestly, Mike, I feel bad that I wasn't more assertive. Maybe it would have done some good."

"No, it wouldn't have. I was completely set in my ways. I wouldn't have listened."

He paused and reached for my hand. "I felt your love, John. I always felt your love. Do you know what that's meant?"

"No."

"More than you'll ever know, carrot brain."

I can't remember the rest of the conversation. I was weeping too hard.

22

On Suffering

LIFE CAN BE HARD, that's for sure. Sometimes it seems as if to hurt is as human as to breathe. The question I ask is this: Is it possible to be aware of our suffering and, at the same time, to maintain our clarity, inner peace, and personal power so that we can respond effectively to the situation? Is it possible to accept the reality of suffering, and also to act to prevent and alleviate as much of it as we can?

I don't think we get there by denying our pain. When we push our suffering away, we fight against the truth of ourselves and this creates dis-ease on many levels. Diet is incredibly important, but one of the great unacknowledged sources of sickness in the modern world is the repression of our feelings and the resultant decline in our capacity for joy and aliveness.

Armoring ourselves in an attempt to keep from experiencing loss depletes us. It's exhausting to hold in our emotions continually. We become passive and resigned—not because we don't care, but because we don't grieve. We shut down because we have allowed our hearts to become so filled with loss that we have no room left to feel. Things like rest, exercise, play, and the releasing of unrealistic expectations are helpful. But sometimes, we really begin to heal only when we learn how to live with our pain, when we become deeply intimate with our suffering, when we learn how to grieve.

This is not always easy to do, but if we try to avoid the pain of facing what is happening, if we seek comfort at any cost, we are left incapable of the love and emotional connection with others that we need in order to be healthy and whole. If we repress our grief, we suffocate our hearts.

We learn early to treat suffering as an enemy to be defeated, to reject what is unpleasant, difficult, or disappointing. Often, we judge ourselves harshly for our woundedness. But healing is not the absence of suffering. Healing is addressing our suffering and allowing it to catalyze responses that bring us to greater wholeness and make us more fully human.

Healing begins with being who we are, with being honest about the reality of ourselves and our world. Compassion requires the courage to face suffering.

The people I've known who've been mentors and lights to my heart and my life have had ways of sharing their joys with other people—and perhaps just as important, their fears and their grief. They recognize that we all have times when we feel overwhelmed and defeated, when we feel terribly alone, when we are tempted to hide in a corner and feel sorry for ourselves. They know we all have dark nights of the soul, and they understand that, at such times, it is necessary to have others to go to, others with whom we can be emotionally vulnerable and honest. In this way, even in the midst of our despair, we are reminded that we are part of a community, that there are others who care about us, and that we are still part of the stream of life. Our grief becomes a source of connection to who we are, to our passion, commitment, courage, and vulnerability.

This is enormously important for us to understand today, because I don't think anyone could become aware of the immensity of what is happening in our world and not feel pain for life and fear for our collective future. We all have our own suffering, of course, our personal losses and disappointments and frustrations. But the pain inside us today goes beyond the personal. It affects each of our individual lives and also something greater. It is the future of life on Earth that now hangs in the balance.

This sorrow belongs to us all. It is in the nature of our times and it is ours to embrace. In the depths of our shared pain, we can also experience our shared caring, our mutual prayers, and the roots of our capacity to act. The pain we feel is the breaking of the shell that encloses our power to respond. Something precious can be born in times like these. In our shared pain, we labor to bring it to birth.

We live now in a time that some call "the great turning," but it is also the great unraveling. In such a time, I believe it is our task to be attentive both to what is dying and what is being born, to what is tragic and what is beautiful. We are called to be unafraid of pain and unafraid of joy, to remember that no feeling is final, and to affirm our power to make a difference.

We are witnesses in our times to wars, destruction, plagues, and pestilence on an almost biblical scale. But what we do with these calamities is up to us. We can let them shatter our resolve and our sense of possibility. Staring into the eyes of history, we can avert our gaze. Or we can use the pain to deepen our commitment to all that is good and life-giving in ourselves and the world.

These are not easy times in which to uphold ourselves and the greater human possibility, nor to feel confident in our collective future. Droughts, raging storms, and rising seas are taking human societies perilously close to the edge. It is profoundly important today that we not give up on ourselves and on one another, that we maintain faith in the higher possibilities of human nature. I, like many, take strength from the reality that, as a species, we have produced people like Dr. Martin Luther King, Jr., Nelson Mandela, and Aung

San Suu Kyi. And I know there are millions of others whose names are not well known who have toiled without acclaim, but whose lives have also demonstrated profound generosity, wisdom, and courage. What I see everywhere I look are ordinary people willing to convert trembling into commitment, brokenness into art, and heartbreak into empathy. In every nook and cranny of this world, there are people willing to confront incalculable odds to restore compassion, hope, and healing.

I think, for example, of the hundreds of thousands of people who have worked day in and day out for decades so that we now stand within a whisker of forever wiping out the last traces of both smallpox and polio from the face of the Earth. And of the hundreds of millions of people worldwide who are endeavoring to create an environmentally sustainable, spiritually fulfilling, and socially just human presence on this planet.

The next time anyone tells you that who you are doesn't matter or that your actions and love are insignificant, here's what they need to know: All who take a stand with their lives on behalf of what they cherish are part of something vast. The struggle for justice is as old as tyranny itself, and the longing for a world guided by love is as old as the human heart.

23

Stronger at the Broken Places

I AM SOMEONE WHO LONGS FOR WORLD PEACE. Perhaps you are, too. And yet every single day our world spends more than $4 billion on war. The last 100 years have been by far the bloodiest in human history.

I support human rights and human dignity. I want every child to grow up healthy and strong. No doubt you do, too. And today, like every day, 20,000 children will die of hunger and in poverty. In the U.S. in 2011, nearly 25 percent of children were living below the poverty line, and more than 45 million Americans were dependent on food stamps in order to eat.

I believe in upholding the brotherhood and sisterhood of all people. I believe in the inherent worth of every human being. And the 400 richest people in the country now control more wealth than 150 million of their fellow Americans. In 2010, twenty-five of the 100 highest-paid U.S. CEOs earned more than their companies paid in federal income tax.

I believe in holding a positive attitude toward life. Yet the rate at which forests are disappearing, coral reefs are deteriorating, the arctic ice cap is melting, and species are becoming extinct is undermining the capacity of the Earth to support human civilization.

I draw strength from my kinship with animals. Some of my best friends have had four legs. Perhaps you, too, have had a relationship with an animal that has enriched you as a human being. And today, almost all of our meat and dairy products come from animals raised under conditions of horrific cruelty.

There are so many kinds of pain and loss in our times. There is growing unemployment and homelessness; there are tsunamis and terrorists, nuclear plant meltdowns, and the threat of world economic collapse. There are things happening in our world today that must make the angels weep.

Here's what I believe. If we're going to face the suffering and destruction of life, and if we want to find a way to be effective and positive in response, we must also be open to the life-affirming powers. Even in the face of the bleakness, we must listen to our creativity and our joy. Even in the midst of so much heartbreaking news, we must dare to dream of peace, possibility, and plenty.

It may sometimes seem as if we are on a planetary death march, and yet we are also living in an age of miracles. Some are so common we often take them for granted. There is the miracle of color and the miracle of music. There is the miracle of tears and the miracle of laughter. There is the miracle of breathing and the miracle of sunsets. There is the miracle of human kindness and the miracle of forgiveness. There is the miracle of people continuing to strive for a happier world even in the face of devastation and grief.

At this very moment, people are learning new ways to communicate, to understand each other, and to resolve conflicts. Right now, people are learning to read, while others are writing poetry, and others are turning degraded lands green again. There are people devoting their lives to ending the sexual abuse of children, and others dedicated to making hunger history. Thanks to the goodwill and efforts of countless people, relationships are growing, new health-giving practices are being discovered, ancient feuds are being overcome, and people are finding ways to restore their connections to the living Earth. Ever-increasing numbers of people are taking responsibility for their health, and giving of themselves so that their families and communities may thrive. We mustn't forget that, at this moment, as in every moment, an ever-growing number of people are working for a better world for themselves and for all children, now and yet to come.

Are we done? Or is it possible that we've only just begun?

Could it be that our despair is not meant to destroy us, but to awaken new life in us?

Yes, there is ugliness—which is why it matters when we bring beauty. Yes, there is great suffering—so let us live with great compassion. Then our wounds can give us depth, empathy, and understanding. Then our hardships can be places where we connect with others and grow.

There are sources of joy here, and we are here to protect and cherish them. We can still make our lives into works of art. We can still create thriving, just, and sustainable ways of life. With all its delusions and broken dreams, our world today is still a place where our hearts can meet and grow wings.

Let us stand for this. Our dreams and prayers are rooted in something greater than the forces of death. Our grief and fury at the world's brutalities are part of our awakening. There is something mysterious taking place in this world that is part of our healing.

Yes, there are forces at work in the human psyche that are destructive and unconscious, but there is also something in us that is wondrous and cares, that touches the infinite and belongs to the sacred.

We are here to live, not merely survive. We are here to express fully and to celebrate the gifts we each have to give to the world, and to receive the gifts that others have to give to us as well.

Let us touch with love the inevitable suffering in our lives and in the lives of those we meet. Let us tend with mercy that which is dying in us and in our world. And let us welcome the new life dawning in each of our souls.

We who are alive, with breath in our bodies and love in our hearts, have so very much to be thankful for. In all that takes place over the course of our lives, may we never lose track of our capacity for gratitude.

Further Reading and Other Resources

THERE ARE SO MANY EXCELLENT BOOKS and other resources available now on all these topics, whether you're interested in reading more about the high personal and planetary costs of industrial food or would like to move toward a more plant-strong diet. The resources listed below just scratch the surface. They are some of my favorites, and the list is growing all the time.

BOOKS

Barnard, Neal, M.D. *Food for Life: How the New Four Food Groups Can Save Your Life*. New York: Three Rivers Press, 1993.

———. *Eat Right, Live Longer: Using the Natural Power of Foods to Age-Proof Your Body*. New York: Three Rivers Press, 1995.

Baur, Gene. *Farm Sanctuary: Changing Hearts and Minds about Animals and Food*. New York: Touchstone, 2008.

Block, Keith I., M.D. *Life Over Cancer: The Block Center Program for Integrative Cancer Treatment*. New York: Bantam Books, 2009.

Brazier, Brendan. *Thrive: The Vegan Nutrition Guide to Optimal Performance in Sports and Life*. Philadelphia, PA: Da Capo Press, 2007.

Campbell, T. Colin, Ph.D. and Thomas M. Campbell II. *The China Study: Startling Implications for Diet, Weight Loss and Long-Term Health*. Dallas, TX: Benbella Books, 2006.

Carr, Kris. *Crazy Sexy Diet: Eat Your Veggies, Ignite Your Spark, and Live Like You Mean It!* Guilford, CT: Globe Pequot Press, 2011.

Davis, Brenda, R.D., and Vesanto Melina, M.S., R.D. *Becoming Vegan: The Complete Guide to Adopting a Plant-Based Diet.* Summertown, TN: Book Publishing Company, 2000.

Eisnitz, Gail. *Slaughterhouse: The Shocking Story of Greed, Neglect, and Inhumane Treatment Inside the U. S. Meat Industry.* Amherst, NY: Prometheus Books, 2007.

Esselstyn, Jr., Caldwell B., M.D. *Prevent and Reverse Heart Disease: The Revolutionary, Scientifically Proven, Nutrition-Based Cure.* New York: Avery, 2007.

Esselstyn, Rip. *The Engine 2 Diet: The Texas Firefighter's 28-Day Save-Your-Life Plan that Lowers Cholesterol and Burns Away the Pounds.* New York: Wellness Central, 2009.

Fitzgerald, Randall. *The Hundred-Year Lie: How to Protect Yourself from the Chemicals That Are Destroying Your Health.* New York: Dutton, 2006.

Foer, Jonathan Safran. *Eating Animals.* New York: Little, Brown and Company, 2009.

Freston. Kathy. *Quantum Wellness: A Practical Guide to Health and Happiness.* New York: Weinstein Books, 2008.

———. *Veganist: Lose Weight, Get Healthy, Change the World.* New York: Weinstein Books, 2011.

Fromartz , Samuel. *Organic, Inc.: Natural Foods and How They Grew.* Orlando, FL: Harcourt, 2006.

Fuhrman, Joel, M.D. *Disease-Proof Your Child: Feeding Kids Right.* New York: St. Martin's Press, 2005.

———. *Eat to Live: The Revolutionary Formula for Fast and Sustained Weight Loss.* New York: Little, Brown and Company, 2003.

Goodall, Jane. *Harvest for Hope: A Guide to Mindful Eating.* New York: Warner Books, 2005.

Halweil, Brian. *Eat Here: Reclaiming Homegrown Pleasures in a Global Supermarket.* New York: W. W. Norton & Company, 2004.

Hever, Julieanna, M.S., R.D., C.P.T. *The Complete Idiot's Guide to Plant-Based Nutrition*. New York: Alpha Books, 2011.

Joy, Melanie. *Why We Love Dogs, Eat Pigs, and Wear Cows: An Introduction to Carnism*. San Francisco: Conari Press, 2010.

Keon, Joseph. *Whitewash: The Disturbing Truth About Cow's Milk and Your Health*. Gabriola Island, BC, Canada: New Society Publishers, 2010.

LaConte, Ellen. *Life Rules: Why So Much Is Going Wrong Everywhere at Once and How Life Teaches Us to Fix It*. Bloomington, IN: iUniverse, 2010.

Lyman, Howard F., and Glen Merzer. *Mad Cowboy: Plain Truth from the Cattle Rancher Who Won't Eat Meat*. New York: Touchstone, 1998.

Lyman, Howard F., Glen Merzer, and Joanna Samorow-Merzer. *No More Bull!: The Mad Cowboy Targets America's Worst Enemy— Our Diet*. New York: Scribner, 2005.

McDougall, John A., M.D. *The McDougal Program for a Healthy Heart: A Lifesaving Approach to Preventing and Treating Heart Disease*. New York: Plume, 1998.

Midkiff, Ken. *The Meat You Eat: How Corporate Farming Has Endangered America's Food Supply*. New York: St. Martin's Press, 2004.

Moore Lappé, Frances, and Anna Lappé. *Hope's Edge: The Next Diet for a Small Planet*. New York: Jeremy P. Tarcher/Putnam, 2002.

Nestle, Marion. *Food Politics: How the Food Industry Influences Nutrition and Health*. Berkeley, CA: University of California Press, 2002.

Niman, Nicolette Hahn. *Righteous Porkchop: Finding a Life and Good Food Beyond Factory Farms*. New York: Collins, 2009.

Ornish, Dean, M.D. *Dr. Dean Ornish's Program for Reversing Heart Disease: The Only System Scientifically Proven to Reverse Heart Disease Without Drugs or Surgery*. New York: Ivy Books, 1990.

Patrick-Goudreau, Colleen. *Color Me Vegan: Maximize Your Nutrient Intake and Optimize Your Health by Eating Antioxidant-Rich, Fiber-Packed, Color-Intense Meals That Taste Great.* Beverly, MA: Fair Winds Press, 2010.

Pollan, Michael. *The Omnivore's Dilemma: A Natural History of Four Meals.* New York: Penguin, 2007.

Robin, Marie-Monique. *The World According to Monsanto: Pollution, Corruption, and the Control of the World's Food Supply.* New York: The New Press, 2008.

Schlosser, Eric. *Fast Food Nation: The Dark Side of the All-American Meal.* New York: Houghton Mifflin Company, 2001.

Servan-Schreiber, David, M.D., Ph.D. *Anticancer, A New Way of Life.* New York: Viking, 2008.

Silverstone, Alicia. *The Kind Diet: A Simple Guide to Feeling Great, Losing Weight, and Saving the Planet.* New York: Rodale, 2009.

Simon, Michele. *Appetite for Profit: How the Food Industry Undermines Our Health and How to Fight Back.* New York: Nation Books, 2006.

Singer, Peter, and Jim Mason. *The Ethics of What We Eat: Why Our Food Choices Matter.* New York: Rodale, 2006.

Smith Jones, Susan. *The Joy Factor: 10 Sacred Practices for Radiant Health.* San Francisco: Conari Press, 2010.

———. *Walking on Air: Your 30-Day Inside and Out Rejuvenation Makeover.* San Francisco, Conari Press, 2011.

Tuttle, Will, Ph.D. *The World Peace Diet: Eating for Spiritual Health and Social Harmony.* New York: Lantern Books, 2005.

DOCUMENTARY FILMS

30 Days (2005–2008). TV series by Morgan Spurlock originally aired on the FX Network.

A Delicate Balance: The Truth (2008). Written and directed by Aaron Scheibner.

Bad Seed: The Truth about Our Food (2006). Written and directed by Timo Nadudvari. Examines the genetic engineering of food from the real-world perspectives of leading scientists, farmers, food-safety advocates, and the victims of genetically engineered products.

Black Gold: Wake Up and Smell the Coffee (2007). Directed by Marc Francis and Nick Francis. An in-depth look at the world of coffee and global trade.

Change Your Food, Change Your Life (2005). DVD produced by Jill Ovnik, president and founder of Vegan-Gal. com. Grocery shopping ideas, smart restaurant choices, and step-by-step recipes for vegan living.

The Corporation (2003). Directed by Mark Achbar and Jennifer Abbott. A documentary that looks at the concept of the corporation throughout recent history up to its present-day dominance.

Death on a Factory Farm (2009). Directed by Tom Simon and Sarah Teale. Documentary about the harrowing treatment of livestock in the United States. Originally aired on HBO March 16, 2009.

Dirt! The Movie (2009). Directed by Bill Benenson, Gene Rosow, and Eleonore Dailly. Narrated by Jamie Lee Curtis. A look at our relationship with dirt and our intimate bond with dirt and the rest of nature.

Fed Up! Genetic Engineering, Industrial Agriculture and Sustainable Alternatives (2006). Directed by Angelo Sacerdote. Humorous but informative facts about the genetic modification of food from scientists, farmers, outspoken activists, and government officials.

Food Fight (2008). Directed by Christopher Taylor. A fascinating look at 20th-century American agricultural policy and food culture and the movement against big agribusiness. Featuring Michael Pollan, Alice Waters, and Marion Nestle.

Food, Inc. (2009). Directed by Robert Kenner. Written by Robert Kenner, Kim Roberts, and Elise Pearlstein. An unflattering look inside America's corporate-controlled food industry.

Food Matters (2008). James Colquhoun and Laurentine Ten Bosch interview world leaders in nutrition and natural healing about the harm we are doing our bodies with improper nutrition and how diet can be used to treat chronic and fatal illnesses.

Forks Over Knives (2011). Written and directed by Lee Fulkerson. Explores how degenerative diseases can be controlled or even reversed by diet.

Fresh (2009). Written by Ana Sofia Joanes. A discussion featuring Will Allen (MacArthur's 2008 Genius Award), sustainable farmer and entrepreneur Joel Salatin, and supermarket owner David Ball that challenges our Walmart-dominated economy.

The Future of Food (2004). Written and directed by Deborah Koons. In-depth investigation into the disturbing truth behind today's unlabeled, patented, genetically-engineered foods.

The Garden (2008). Written and directed by Scott Hamilton Kennedy. The story of the largest community garden in the United States, now threatened by bulldozers.

Inside Job (2010). Written and directed by Charles Ferguson, narrated by Matt Damon. Takes a closer look at what brought about the financial meltdown.

King Corn (2007). Directed by Aaron Woolf. Feature documentary that questions the assumptions of modern agribusiness and raises troubling questions about our food industry and government food policy.

Meat the Truth (2008). Written and directed by Karen Soeters. An examination of intensive livestock production that shows it generates more greenhouse gas emissions worldwide than fossil-fueled vehicles.

McLibel: The Story of Two People Who Wouldn't Say McSorry (2005). Produced and directed by Franny Armstrong. The story of two ordinary people who stood up to the multinational power of McDonald's in the biggest corporate PR disaster in history.

The Power of Community: How Cuba Survived Peak Oil (2009). Directed by Faith Morgan. An exploration of Cuba's transition from oil-dependent farms and plantations and a reliance on fossil-fuel-based pesticides and fertilizers, to small organic farms and urban gardens.

Processed People (2009). Directed by Jeff Nelson. Written by Sabrina Nelson. A factual, hard-hitting commentary on diet and health.

The Real Dirt on Farmer John (2006). Directed by Taggart Siegel. Epic tale of a maverick Midwestern farmer who transforms his farm amid a failing economy, vicious rumors, and arson.

The Story of Stuff (2007). Directed by Louis Fox. Animated short that questions our culture of consumption and opens a serious dialog about our reliance on "stuff. "

Super Size Me (2004). Written and directed by Morgan Spurlock. A personal exploration of the health consequences of a diet consisting solely of McDonald's food.

Vanishing of the Bees (2009). Directed by George Langworthy and Maryam Henein. A study of the sudden disappearance of honey bees caused by the poorly understood phenomenon known as Colony Collapse Disorder (CCD).

The Witness (2000). Directed by James LaVeck and Jenny Stein. The story of a man who feared and avoided animals most of his life, until a life-changing experience inspired him to advocate for the rescue of abandoned animals.

The World According to Monsanto (2008). Directed by Marie-Monique Robin. A documentary that traces a wide range of controversies involving the use and promotion of genetically-modified seeds, polychlorinated biphenyls, and bovine growth hormone.

About the Author

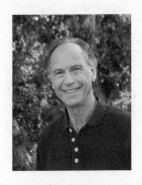

Groomed to follow in the footsteps of his father, founder of the Baskin-Robbins empire, John Robbins chose a different path for himself, becoming a social activist and fierce advocate for plant-strong diets and compassionate living. John Robbins is the author of *The Food Revolution*, *Diet for a New America*, *Reclaiming Our Health*, and *The New Good Life*. His life and work have been featured on the PBS special *Diet for a New America*, and he has won numerous awards for his pioneering work, including the Rachel Carson Award, the Albert Schweitzer Humanitarian Award, the Peace Abbey's Courage of Conscience Award, and Green America's Lifetime Achievement Award.

He lives with his family in the Santa Cruz Mountains.

Visit him at *www.johnrobbins.info*.

John Robbins' Website

You are invited to visit *www.johnrobbins.info* for tools, leading-edge information, and a comprehensive resource guide to help you live and share the message of this book.

When you visit, you'll find:

- Organizations, websites, books, films, and tools
- Information about events with John Robbins and how to contact him
- Articles by and videos featuring John Robbins
- Questions and answers on important topics

Please visit *www.johnrobbins.info*.

To Our Readers

Conari Press, an imprint of Red Wheel/Weiser, publishes books on topics ranging from spirituality, personal growth, and relationships to women's issues, parenting, and social issues. Our mission is to publish quality books that will make a difference in people's lives—how we feel about ourselves and how we relate to one another. We value integrity, compassion, and receptivity, both in the books we publish and in the way we do business.

Our readers are our most important resource, and we appreciate your input, suggestions, and ideas about what you would like to see published.

Visit our website *www.redwheelweiser.com* where you can learn about our upcoming books and free downloads, and be sure to go to *www.redwheelweiser.com/newsletter/* to sign up for newsletters and exclusive offers.

You can also contact us at *info@redwheelweiser.com*.

Conari Press
an imprint of Red Wheel/Weiser, LLC
665 Third Street, Suite 400
San Francisco, CA 94107